Fit to Deliver

AN INNOVATIVE PRENATAL AND POSTPARTUM FITNESS PROGRAM

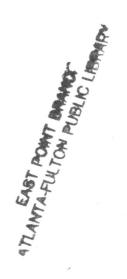

Fit to Deliver

AN INNOVATIVE PRENATAL AND
POSTPARTUM FITNESS PROGRAM

by
Karen Nordahl, M.D.
Carl Petersen, B.P.E., B.Sc. (PT)
Renée Minges Jeffreys, M.Sc.

Hartley
& Marks
PUBLISHERS

Published by
HARTLEY & MARKS PUBLISHERS INC.
P.O. Box 147   3661 West Broadway
Point Roberts, WA   Vancouver, B.C.
98281   V6R 2B8

LIBRARY OF CONGRESS CATALOGING-IN-PUBLICATION DATA

Nordahl, Karen M., 1963–
    Fit to deliver : an innovative prenatal and postpartum fitness program
by Karen M. Nordahl, Carl Petersen, Renée Minges Jeffreys.
        p. cm.
    Previously published in 2000.
    Includes bibliographical references and index.
    ISBN 0-88179-208-x (pbk.)   —ISBN 978088179208X
      1. Physical fitness for pregnant women.   2. Postnatal care.   I. Petersen,
Carl, 1956–   II. Jeffreys, Renée Minges, 1971–   III. Title.
        RG558.7.N67 2004
        618.2'44—dc22   2004023640

Printed in Canada.

ACKNOWLEDGMENTS

We would like to thank our families and friends for their support during this process. We'd also like to thank the researchers who ask the questions and find the answers that we can then apply in our professional lives.

This book is dedicated to all the participants of our fitness classes that we have had the pleasure to work with over the years. It is your demand for knowledge that has fueled our passion.

Karen, Carl and Renée would like to give a special thank-you to
Niki Denroche, Personal Trainer
Shanna Stevens, Physical Therapist
Sarah Arscott, BSc HKin and
Martha Sirdevan, Physical Therapist for reviewing key sections.

Thanks also to Patricia Chuey, MSc, RDN for writing the section on Nutrition; Jody Timlick, RN for writing the section on Relaxation; and Nina Nittinger, Dipl. KFFR/Sports Mgt. for writing the section on Nordic Walking. A special thank-you to all the very patient exercise models: Carolyn, Cheryl, Cindy, Danielle, Heidi, Joanne, Lisa and Patricia.

CONTENTS

Preface

A physician, a physical therapist and an exercise physiologist may seem like odd bedfellows. Yet, our combined knowledge offers an innovative and intuitive path to wellness during a complex and exciting period in a woman's life—pregnancy.

Advances in knowledge about fitness and pregnancy have meant women are no longer considered to be in "confinement," but rather in a natural stage of life. Prenatal and postpartum women can and should take active measures to ensure optimum health, for their own benefit and that of their baby, by engaging in basic fitness routines.

We've brought together three different but interconnected perspectives to produce a benchmark health and fitness resource for pregnant and postpartum women. This book relies on the latest scientific research, and on the practical knowledge of health and fitness professionals who work with women throughout their pregnancies.

The goal of *Fit to Deliver* is two-fold: to give women the ability to modify their existing fitness program (or, for those new to exercise, to start a program); and to go one step further by offering state-of-the-art training techniques to better prepare for delivery and the postpartum period.

Fit to Deliver exercises focus on "functional" activity, or the types of activities that train the muscles used on a regular basis. These exercises will be helpful to women throughout their childbearing years. The benefits gained by learning how to exercise safely and effectively will last a lifetime.

How to Use This Book

Please read chapters 1 and 2 before you begin so that you are aware of safety concerns and fitness guidelines that will help you and your baby get the most out of the Fit to Deliver program.

This book is designed to give you flexibility in choosing your own fitness program, tailored to your fitness level and your stage of pregnancy.

If you're looking for more variety or you require a more tailored approach to suit your needs, you can start fresh by designing your own program. All the ingredients are here for you to develop routines that will fit your schedule and help you reach your goals.

Chapter 3, "The Core," focuses on the postural changes in your body during pregnancy and the exercises that will help your body comfortably adjust and thrive during its 40-week (plus) marathon. Once you have mastered the "Five on the Floor," which are essential to maintaining core strength, you can try the other core exercises and add the ones you're most comfortable with.

Chapter 5 contains a variety of exercises to choose from in a warm-up, stretching and cooldown routine. Be sure to adequately warm up before and cool down after your workout, and make it a priority to incorporate stretching exercises into each workout.

During a week, be sure to include cardio, strength, balance and relaxation exercises in a well-rounded program (remember that they don't all have to be done in the same day). If you have questions, make sure you consult a qualified fitness professional.

The key to achieving the greatest benefit from a prenatal fitness program is consistency: aim to exercise for 30 to 60 minutes, 4 to 6 days a week, throughout your pregnancy.

Of course, many of these exercises can be done as you go about your day-to-day routine, and remember that some exercise is always better than none. Do what you can, when you can, and keep it fun!

Karen Nordahl, MD
Carl Petersen, BPE, BSC (PT)
Renée M. Jeffreys, MSc

> **NOTE**
> *The core exercises are the foundation of the Fit to Deliver program and should be done daily.*

Exercise Benefits for Mother and Baby

Benefits to the pregnant woman

Women who perform aerobic exercise for 45-minute sessions, at least 5 times per week, will receive the majority of the benefits listed below. The exercise must be weight bearing (i.e., not swimming) and aerobic for benefits to be appreciated. There has not been any research published to date on the currently popular forms of prenatal exercise such as yoga or Pilates (Clapp, 2002).

Women who exercise at a mild to moderate intensity, at least three times per week, will experience an improvement in their well-being, reduced constipation, fewer leg cramps and a quicker return to pre-pregnancy weight when compared to their non-exercising counterparts (ACOG, 2002; Clapp, 2002).

- Reduced risk of developing gestational diabetes (especially in women with a body mass index—BMI—greater than 33)
- Reduced risk of developing pregnancy-induced hypertension (high blood pressure)
- Fewer obstetric interventions (vacuum extraction, forceps)
- Reduction in the "active stage" of labor (the time from 4 cm to 10 cm dilation)
- Research has suggested that the incidence of caesarean section may be lower in women who exercise during pregnancy

- Increase in maternal well-being—you will have more energy and sleep more soundly
- Increased sense of control over your pregnancy and your changing body
- Improved self image
- Quicker return to pre-pregnancy weight
- Decreased incidence of loss of bladder control during pregnancy and postpartum
- Reduction in bone density loss while breastfeeding
- Reduction in common pregnancy complaints such as hemorrhoids, constipation, leg cramps, back pain, etc.

Benefits to babies

Most of the following benefits to babies are achieved with moderate exercise programs.

1. Infants have less body fat at birth. Some early research suggests that the benefits of lower body fat may translate into a reduction in the incidence of heart disease and diabetes in adulthood.
2. Infants are less cranky and less likely to have colic.
3. Children have greater neurodevelopmental scores in oral language and motor areas when tested at age 5.

Common pregnancy complaints that improve with exercise

Your body undergoes enormous changes to accommodate your growing baby and prepare you for birth. You have to deal with your enlarging abdomen, bigger breasts, incontinence and an aching back. Exercising before you are pregnant may reduce your chances of developing some of the aches and pains that go along with this wonderful time in your life. Exercising during pregnancy may actually help alleviate them altogether.

- *Lower back pain:* due to the extra weight you are carrying, poor posture and pelvic widening. It may be alleviated by pelvic and core exercises. It is important that you "check" your posture regularly, and maintain proper form when lifting and carrying.

- *Upper back pain:* due to the rounding of your shoulders from extra breast weight. Make sure you perform pectoral muscle stretches and shoulder shrugs, and check your posture.

- *Carpal tunnel syndrome:* usually caused by the extra swelling that comes with water retention and weight gain. It may be reduced by wrist circles and finger squeezes. You may want to contact your caregiver for advice on wrist splints.

- *Leg cramps:* usually caused by dehydration or calcium deficiency. Gentle calf stretches may be helpful, but do not stretch too aggressively. Talk to your caregiver about possibly increasing your calcium intake.

- *Leg swelling:* caused by water retention. Ankle rotations are helpful.

- *Incontinence of urine:* caused by the weight of your baby on your bladder, and the hormonal changes that cause pelvic widening. Pelvic floor and core exercises are helpful.

Myths of Exercise and Pregnancy

Until just a few generations ago, women were confined to the house during pregnancy. (Your caregiver may still refer to your due date as an EDC, or "estimated date of confinement.") It was believed that an active pregnant woman would divert blood away from her growing fetus and toward her exercising muscles, resulting in a smaller baby. As society evolved and women began to take a more active role in the community, confinement during pregnancy became impractical. Moreover, the first studies on this subject, in 1970, demonstrated that moderate exercise is safe and, in fact, beneficial in a normal, healthy pregnancy.

Misconceptions about exercise during pregnancy

1. Exercise during pregnancy can increase your risk of miscarriage.

This has not been demonstrated in any research. There is a slightly increased risk of miscarriage if you overheat during the first trimester, but this is true whether you exercise or not. Therefore, it is very important that you do not overheat during your exercise sessions.

2. Exercise during pregnancy will make your infant smaller at birth.

Moderate exercise during a normal, healthy pregnancy does not have this effect.

3. Exercise during pregnancy may cause you to go into labor prematurely.

This has not been reproduced in large studies. Pregnant exercising women do give birth about nine days sooner than their non-exercising counterparts, but this is not considered premature labor.

4. *It is not safe to start an exercise program when you are pregnant.*

Research has demonstrated that it is quite safe to begin a low-intensity exercise program in the first to mid-second trimesters.

Fit to Deliver Philosophy
Our Vision

We have a vision that someday, for herself and her newborn, every pregnant woman will choose to follow a planned fitness program before, during and after pregnancy.

The Fit to Deliver program follows three principles:

Prevention

Participating in a regular exercise program can help to prevent many common pregnancy complaints such as back pain, diastasis recti (separation of the abdominal muscles) and a weak pelvic floor. Exercising during pregnancy has also been found to reduce the incidence of gestational diabetes and pregnancy-induced hypertension.

Preparation

The Fit to Deliver program will help you prepare for the rigors of labor by strengthening the muscles needed during labor, the "baby pushers." Labor is probably one of the more intense activities that you will experience, and preparing for it physically will give you an advantage. Once the baby arrives you will have to be ready to care for your infant, and all the strength that you have gained or maintained participating in a prenatal fitness program will be useful.

Restoration

After the baby has arrived, the time spent exercising during pregnancy will make it easier for you to regain your pre-pregnancy shape, strength and fitness level.

Before You Begin

Before You Begin the Fit to Deliver Program

Contraindications to Exercising

1. Ensure your healthcare provider is aware that you are exercising during your pregnancy.
2. Fill out the PARmed-X screening form with your caregiver. (The form is found on the Canadian Society for Exercise Physiology website at www.csep.ca)
3. Listen to your body—now is the time to maintain, not increase, your fitness level.
4. Read carefully and follow the ACOG safe exercise guidelines summarized below.

Remember: Your healthcare provider is the best source of information about your individual pregnancy.

The following guidelines are adapted from the American College of Obstetricians and Gynecologists (ACOG) publication on exercise during pregnancy (2002).

Absolute Contraindications to Aerobic Exercise During Pregnancy

You should not exercise during pregnancy if you have any of the following:

- Significant heart disease
- Lung disease (for example, severe asthma)
- Incompetent cervix/cerclage
- Multiple gestation (twins or triplets) at risk for premature labor
- Persistent second or third trimester bleeding
- Placenta previa after 26 weeks' gestation (a condition where the placenta covers the cervix)
- Premature labor during the current pregnancy
- Ruptured membranes
- Preeclampsia/pregnancy-induced hypertension (high blood pressure)

Relative Contraindications to Aerobic Exercise During Pregnancy

You may exercise with extra supervision if you have any of the following:

- Severe anemia
- Unevaluated maternal cardiac arrhythmia (irregular heart beat)
- Chronic bronchitis
- Poorly controlled type I diabetes (insulin dependent)
- Extreme morbid obesity
- Extreme underweight (BMI less than 12)
- History of extremely sedentary lifestyle
- Intrauterine growth retardation, or a baby that is "small for dates," in current pregnancy
- Poorly controlled hypertension
- Orthopedic limitations
- Poorly controlled seizure disorder
- Poorly controlled hyperthyroidism
- Heavy smoker

Guidelines for Exercising While Pregnant

The following is a summary of the revised ACOG guidelines (2002).

1. In the absence of contraindications (above) pregnant women are encouraged to engage in 30 minutes or more of moderate exercise on most, if not all, days of the week. A woman should always check with her caregiver before beginning an exercise program.

2. After the first trimester, pregnant women should avoid supine positions during exercise. Motionless standing should also be avoided.

3. Participation in a wide variety of recreational activities is safe. However, any activity with a high risk for falling or abdominal trauma should be avoided. Examples are ice hockey, soccer, basketball and vigorous racquet sports.

4. Scuba diving should only be performed under a physician's direction.

5. Exertion at altitudes up to 6000 feet appears to be safe. Engaging in physical activities at higher altitudes carries a risk of hypoxemia.

When to Terminate Exercise While Pregnant

Discontinue your exercise program and seek medical advice if you experience any of the following:

- Vaginal bleeding
- Dyspnea (shortness of breath) prior to exertion
- Dizziness
- Headache
- Chest pain
- Muscle weakness
- Calf pain or swelling (deep vein thrombosis must be ruled out)
- Preterm labor
- Decreased fetal movement
- Amniotic fluid leakage

General Recommendations

In the 2002 ACOG Committee Opinion on Exercise during Pregnancy and the Postpartum Period, ACOG stated that pregnant women can adopt the same exercise recommendation made by the Centers for Disease Control (CDC) and the American College of Sports Medicine (ACSM) for the non-pregnant population. This recommendation is 30 or more* accumulated minutes of moderate physical activity on all or most days of the week. As a rule of thumb, based on guidelines for the non-pregnant population, cardiovascular training should be done a minimum of three days per week, strength training a minimum of one day per week, and flexibility training in conjunction with cardiovascular or strength training.

* The recommendation of 30 minutes of moderate activity comes from the Surgeon General's Report on Physical Activity. In 2002, the Institutes of Medicine issued a statement indicating that research had shown the need for 60 minutes daily of moderate physical activity, and we recommend following this revised guideline.

Exercise and High-Risk Pregnancy

Exercise is a safe addition to a normal, healthy pregnancy. But what happens if your pregnancy has complications? What if your blood pressure increases or you are carrying twins? The guidelines below will assist you in modifying your exercise program. With pregnancies that are high risk you must receive approval from your caregiver before continuing to exercise. Any condition listed under the relative or absolute contraindications should be reviewed with your caregiver.

Do not continue your aerobic exercise program if:

- You are having twins and the doctor has told you that you are at risk for early labor
- You have vaginal bleeding
- You have placenta previa and are past your 26th week (the placenta covers the cervix, confirmed by obstetrical ultrasound)
- You have high blood pressure as a result of your pregnancy
- You have premature labor in this pregnancy
- You have an incompetent cervix (a cervix that dilates prematurely, sometimes managed with a "stitch" in the cervix)
- Your membranes are ruptured
- You have a medical condition that would preclude you from exercising when you are not pregnant (for example, heart or lung disease).

Note that the guidelines suggest termination of aerobic exercise. With your caregiver's approval, you may be able to do some stretching or bed-based exercises.

Modify your exercise program if:

- You have intrauterine growth retardation in this pregnancy (small for dates)
- You have any other medical condition that would preclude you from exercising while not pregnant.

Modification of your program could include a reduction in the frequency and/or intensity of your workouts. These modifications are extremely individualized, so you must discuss your condition with your caregiver or fitness professional.

Finding a Qualified Prenatal Fitness Professional

Fitness Professionals

It is important to work with a qualified fitness professional during your pregnancy. Currently there is no national certification or licensing program, so anyone can claim to be a "personal trainer." Look for an instructor with a degree in a physical activity–related field, such as exercise science, exercise physiology or physical fitness/education.

There are several national certifications. The American College of Sports Medicine (ACSM) is considered the gold standard. Others include the American Council on Exercise (ACE), the National Association of Sports Medicine (NASM) and the National Strength Training Association (NSTA).

Instructors should also have experience working with pregnant women. The Fit to Deliver, Moms in Motion and Healthy Moms programs are well-respected prenatal education courses that professionals should have, in addition to the ones listed above.

Physical Therapists

Some physical therapists (PT) work as both rehabilitation and fitness professionals. Physical therapists are licensed by the state. Rules vary by state as to whether you can see a PT directly or if you must have a referral from a physician; check with your insurance provider to determine the rules in your state. Insurance covers physical therapy required for rehabilitation purposes, but not for general fitness purposes.

Steps to a Successful Fit to Deliver Program

This section will give you an overview of the guidelines associated with exercise and pregnancy. This overview is not exhaustive and you should review the entire book before you start your exercise program.

Invest in Good Athletic Clothing

In order to be comfortable and prevent injury during exercise, two pieces of athletic clothing are a must:

- Sports bra: During pregnancy, breasts become larger and more sensitive. Having a supportive sports bra can make exercise more comfortable during both high- and low-impact activities. You may need to purchase a larger bra as your pregnancy progresses. Fit to Deliver recommends Mothers in Motion® exercise wear.
- Shoes: Your feet bear the brunt of your pregnancy, and a good pair of athletic shoes can help to prevent joint pain. Feet may swell or even increase in size, so make sure your shoes are not restrictive. If they become confining, replace them with a bigger size. Reputable athletic shoe stores can help you to fit your feet properly.

Listen to Your Body

- Now is not the time to push yourself. If you feel overly fatigued take a break, or spend extra time stretching or just warming up. Discontinue your program if you have muscle pain, abdominal cramping, bleeding or fluid leakage.
- Plan rest days into your exercise program, and take adequate rest between workouts and within the workout (between sets of exercises).
- Mix up your activities, doing strength training one day and aerobic/cardio training the next. This gives the muscles time to recover between workouts.
- If you experience any pain in your joints, muscles or otherwise while exercising you have probably done too much, too soon, too fast or too often.

Exercise Smarts

Set up a schedule that includes the following principles:

- Do some form of exercise at least 4 to 6 times per week, depending on your trimester and fitness level.
- Adjust your daily activity or exercise based on how you feel that day.
- You can modify your workout by changing the length of time (total time, or number of reps), the intensity (speed or weight) or frequency (number of days per week).

Watch Your Diet and Hydration

- Exercise burns calories, which you must replace to ensure adequate nutrition for your growing baby. Exercise should not be used as a means to limit weight gain.
- Pregnant women typically are told to consume an additional 300 calories per hour

of exercise, but this has been found to be excessive. It is better to eat to appetite, and to make positive food choices.

- Stay well hydrated, as dehydration has been found to be a precursor to premature labor. Drink an extra 8 ounces of water for every 20 minutes of aerobic activity. Be sure to drink before and after your workout. Drink to thirst.

Keep It Fun!

Carrying out a prenatal exercise program and continuing after delivery is one of the best lifestyle and health choices that you will ever make. Engaging in physical activity is a highly effective means of managing weight, promoting health and reducing stress. Getting in the habit of doing some exercise daily, regardless of the level of fitness produced, will help set the trend for your improved lifestyle.

Whether your goal is simply to maintain fitness or to improve it, you need consistency and commitment. With today's fast-paced lifestyles it can be inconvenient or downright impossible to find the time to work out, and staying motivated can be especially difficult during the cold, wet winter months. Following are some ideas to ensure that your workouts are productive, rewarding and, above all, fun.

General Trimester Guidelines
First trimester (0 to 12 weeks)

- If you were previously active, you can continue your exercise program.
- If you were previously inactive, begin by consulting a qualified health or exercise professional. Walking is an easy and effective start.
- All women should look to accumulate a minimum of 30 to 60 minutes of moderate physical activity on all or most days of the week, if there are no medical or obstetrical reasons precluding exercise.
- Stay well hydrated and don't become fatigued or overheated.

Second trimester (13 to 27 weeks)

- If you were previously active, you should maintain your exercise program. Research has shown that consistency is the key to reaping the benefits of exercise during pregnancy (Clapp, 1994; Clapp, 2002).
- The baby leaves the protection of the pelvis, so modify or avoid sports that could result in abdominal trauma.
- Now is often the time that non-exercisers begin an exercise program. If you choose to start an exercise program, do so with a qualified health or exercise professional.
- Do not exercise on your back for more than 30 seconds.

> ### TIPS FROM THE TEAM
>
> *Do Not Monitor Heart Rate*
> Heart rate was abandoned as a measure of exercise intensity during pregnancy in 1994. Instead, use your Rate of Perceived Exertion or the talk test guidelines.
>
> *Always Fire the Core and Sustain*
> During all exercise and activities try maintaining tension in your inner core muscles (pelvic floor and transversus abdominis).

• Stay well hydrated and don't become fatigued or overheated.

Third trimester
(28 weeks to delivery)

• Do not exercise on your back for more than 30 seconds.
• Listen very closely to your body during this stage.
• Exercising at this point becomes increasingly difficult. So as not to lose all the good you have done, stay as close to your second trimester routine as possible. Although you may be tempted to abandon your fitness program, decreasing physical activity now may result in a heavier baby and more discomforts.
• Stay well hydrated and don't become fatigued or overheated.

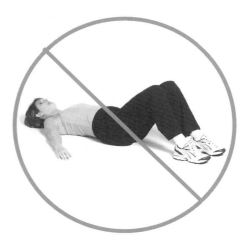

Do not exercise on your back for more than 30 seconds.

TIPS FROM THE TEAM

List Your Reasons For Exercising
Create a list of reasons why you want to improve your health and that of your baby by exercising consistently. Keep a pen and paper handy for several days and jot down ideas that come to mind. Make the list detailed and review it each month or when your motivation is waning.

Put Exercise on Your "To Do" List
Four to six times a week, book yourself an appointment to exercise. Reserve a time slot for working out and don't let anything interfere. Choose a time that is convenient so you will be more likely to keep your exercise appointment.

Stay Committed
Inform everyone of your exercise time. If you are approached to do something else during your designated exercise session, invite that person to join you in working out or to reschedule the appointment.

Plan Ahead
If you plan on working out first thing in the morning, set out your exercise clothes the night before, or have your gym bag packed for the next evening's class. The easier you make it to exercise the more likely you will do it, especially when other demands arise that may tempt you to put it off for later.

Commute with a Workout
Early in your pregnancy try walking or walk-jogging to or from work. This exercise can be done in any weather; just keep an extra set of clothes at your office if it has a shower, or find a fitness club nearby where you can get showered and changed. Varying the route and alternating between a steady pace and easy intervals (a little faster) for short periods of time keeps your workout fresh.

Minimize Quantity, Emphasize Quality
Forget about the "no pain, no gain" mentality. Training or exercising shouldn't be painful, and if it is you are working too hard or too often, failing to rest your body between sessions or wearing the wrong shoes. By emphasizing quality (maintaining good form, completing the full range of motion) you can decrease the amount of time you spend exercising and still get an effective workout.

Exercise Splitting
If one day you can't find 60 minutes for a workout, try exercising in two 30-minute sessions or four 15-minute sessions. These short sessions are preferable to skipping your workout altogether.

Do It Inside
If you can't bear to brave the elements, move your workout indoors. Try exercising on a treadmill, stairclimber, elliptical trainer, exercise bike or rowing machine. Varying your routine produces a good cross-training effect and helps alleviate boredom.

Work on Your Weaknesses
If you are already a strong walker, try alternating walking with stationary cycling or stairclimbing. If flexibility is a problem for you, ensure you spend adequate time stretching. If stability, strength or balance are your weaknesses, do more strength and stabilization drills. Give yourself an honest assessment of your exercise habits, strengths and weaknesses. Your exercise physiologist, physical therapist or personal trainer can help you identify problem areas and individualize your program.

When doing strength work, concentrate on the weakest area first and when stretching, always begin with the tightest muscle groups.

TIPS FROM THE TEAM

Walking Workouts

Walking is an ideal workout during pregnancy. It's easy, carries virtually no risk of injury and requires no special equipment except good, supportive shoes and comfortable clothes. Walking is pleasurable alone or with a companion or group. Few walking devotees ever get bored and quit. Walking to the store or to and from work can be a great break from the day's routine. After-meal walks help promote digestion.

Partner Up

Exercising with others will help motivate you when you're feeling lazy. Be sure to choose your exercise partner wisely – pick someone who is reliable, motivated and committed. Try meeting with friends for an exercise date once or twice a week, or join an exercise class. If you make yourself accountable to an exercise partner you will be less likely to skip your workout.

Reward Yourself

Pay yourself to exercise. Put a few dollars in a piggy bank every time you exercise, and at the end of the month spend this money on something you normally wouldn't buy for yourself.

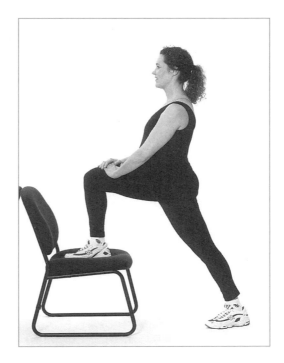

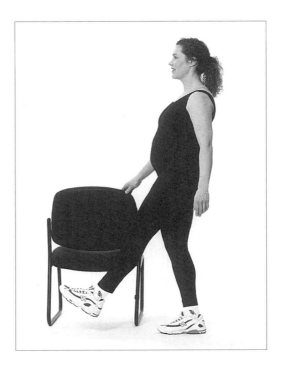

The Core: Your Key to a Healthy Pregnancy

Background on the Core

The key to the Fit to Deliver program is the core. This is not a simple concept and you may need to review this section several times before it all becomes clear, but stick with it! Mastering the concept of core stability will improve your fitness exponentially.

We usually think of the core as the abdominal and lower back muscles, but for the purposes of this book consider the pelvic floor and core (PF-Core) as working as an integrated cylindrical unit. You may visualize this unit as the core of an apple, not simply the outside skin. By focusing on the core you can reduce back pain and improve the ability to perform daily chores during and after pregnancy with much greater ease. Exercises for the PF-Core should be included in all workouts and throughout the day with activities of daily living.

Anatomy of the Core Cylinder (The Apple Core)

The core cylinder consists of many bones, joints and muscles.

Internal Core Muscles

The lumbopelvic core is made up of four muscles that are effective at stabilizing the low back and pelvis: transversus abdominis, pelvic floor, multifidus and diaphragm. Collectively, these muscles form a corset around the lumbar spine and pelvis providing a flexible cylinder of support. Proper function and recruitment of each of these muscles is essential for stability; inadequate function compromises the entire core.

The Bones and Joints

The bones consist of the vertebral column (spine) and its 24 flexible vertebrae, which are classified into three regions based on their structure and function (cervical, thoracic and lumbar). The base of the core cylinder is formed by the lumbar spine and

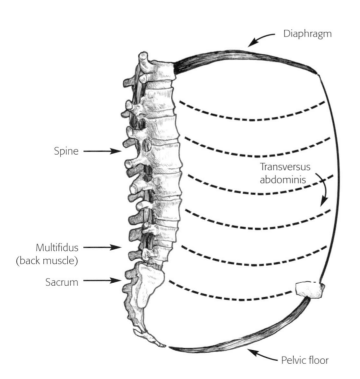

Core cylinder (adapted from Lee, 2000).

pelvis. The pelvis is made up of three irregularly shaped bones that are strongly connected and surround our reproductive organs. Above the pelvis are five lumbar vertebrae. These large vertebrae provide the muscles and ligaments with strong attachment sites. Farther up the spine is the thoracic region (including the ribs) which has limited mobility and is designed to protect the lungs and heart. At the top of the spine is the cervical region which is designed for mobility.

The sacroiliac joint connects the sacrum to the pelvis, and it transfers the weight or load from the trunk to the lower extremities. A small amount of movement is always possible at this joint, but its flexibility increases during pregnancy due to the hormone relaxin which helps prepare for the baby's passage through the birth canal. The front of the pelvis is joined in the midline by the pubic symphysis, which is a cartilaginous joint that can become more flexible and possibly separate (a condition called diastasis symphysis) during pregnancy. The hip joint connects the pelvis and the femur. The hip is a ball and socket-shaped joint that allows for a high degree of movement.

The Muscles
Abdominal Muscles
There are four abdominal muscles: the transversus abdominis, rectus abdominis, internal obliques and external obliques. The transversus abdominis acts like a sling across the lower abdomen, running horizontally from one side of the pelvis to the other. The rectus abdominis is a long muscle that originates at the ribcage and sternum and inserts into the pubic bone. It is wider at its origin, where it fans out to attach, and narrower at its point of insertion. The internal and external obliques run between the ribs on an oblique angle, the internal obliques

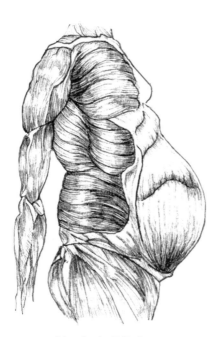

Muscles in 3-D view.

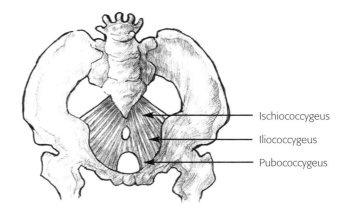

Ischiococcygeus

Iliococcygeus

Pubococcygeus

Pelvic floor muscles.

angling upward and the external obliques angling downward.

The Pelvic Floor Muscles:
The Bottom of the Cylinder

The pelvic floor is made up of a sling of three muscles—pubococcygeus, iliococcygeus and ischiococcygeus—that connects the pubic bone at the front to the coccyx (tailbone) and ischial tuberosities (sitting bones) at the back. This sling serves as a "floor" that is a vital support structure for the contents of the pelvis and abdomen, including your bladder, uterus and bowel. As your baby grows, the extra weight on the pelvic floor muscles makes them work harder. It is very important to keep these muscles strong to prevent problems such as incontinence or uterine prolapse.

What can cause pelvic floor weakness?
- Constipation (i.e., excessive straining to empty your bowel)

- Persistent heavy lifting
- Excessive coughing causing repetitive straining
- Childbirth, particularly following delivery of a large baby or prolonged pushing during delivery
- Changes in hormonal levels at menopause may further weaken damaged muscles.

Transversus Abdominis (TA)

The transversus abdominis (TA) is the innermost abdominal muscle that connects to the spine at the back and wraps around the trunk to meet its counterpart in the front. It has a large area of attachment to the lower six ribs and the top of the entire pelvis. When transversus abdominis contracts it causes a slight narrowing of the waist and drawing in of the lower abdomen, something like a tight corset. It functions to stiffen the spine and stabilize the pelvis prior to movements of the arms and legs. Thus, in people who use proper stabilization strategies the transversus abdominis is frequently active at a low level throughout the day. This is what you will want to achieve with the Fit to Deliver program "Fire the Core and Sustain" (McKechnie & Celebrini, 1999).

During pregnancy the pelvic floor, TA and other abdominal muscles become very stretched and their ability to stabilize and support the lower back and pelvis is reduced. The pelvic floor must support an ever-increasing weight as your baby and uterus grow. In addition, the internal fascial support system for the uterus and bladder can become stretched as well. During a vaginal delivery, the anterior pelvic floor becomes even more stretched and occasionally torn or cut (during an episiotomy). If you

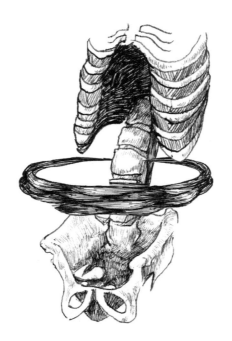

Transversus abdominis
(adapted from Celebrini, 2001).

have had a caesarean section the pelvic floor is preserved, but the surgery causes further trauma to the abdominal wall.

After your delivery the function of the TA and the anterior pelvic floor is not immediately restored and your stabilization mechanisms may not be as efficient as they need to be. Repeated bending as you care for your newborn and undertake your activities of daily living places stress on the pelvic and lumbar joints. This is why exercising the muscles of the pelvic floor and core throughout your pregnancy and soon after delivery is very important for your health.

What Can Be Done?

All women should regularly exercise the pelvic floor and core muscles. During pregnancy this becomes especially important. Strong pelvic floor muscles can prevent or minimize embarrassing urine leaks when laughing, sneezing or lifting heavy loads. Kegel exercises are the most common method of working these muscles, and when done consistently even weak muscles can be strengthened to perform effectively again.

Finding Your Core Muscles

Isolating the Transversus Abdominis (TA)

Now that you understand where the core muscles are located and what they do, let's focus on how we exercise them throughout the childbearing years and beyond. Curl up with this important section of the book and find each muscle group individually first. After you locate the muscles you will be able to work them as a unit. Don't get frustrated; for some women this is an entirely new way to train.

The transversus abdominis can be felt or palpated on the lower part of the abdomen just inside the anterior superior iliac spine of the pelvis. Place two fingers on the crest of your pelvic bone and move them slightly toward your belly button. When transversus abdominis contracts, a light tension can be felt (you Fire the Core and Sustain). If the abdomen pushes out or bulges or the back flattens, you are using the wrong muscles. When this happens, not only are the wrong muscles firing, but you are in effect turning off the transversus abdominis. If you are having trouble finding the TA, pretend you are trying to stop the flow of urine and it will fire automatically. This is because when you contract one part of the core (the pelvic floor in this case), the other parts of the core contract synergistically, or at the same time.

Fire the Core and Sustain (lying supine)

- Lie on your back with your head supported, knees comfortably bent and feet flat on the floor.
- Picture the abdomen either as a clock or as compass points N, S, E, W with 12:00 or N just below the breastbone, 6:00 or S just above the pubis and the other points just inside the prominent front pelvic bones.
- Keep 12:00 (N) and 6:00 (S) in the same position (i.e., maintain a lengthened spine) and draw 9:00 and 3:00 (W and E) apart. Imagine the TA pulling the fascia of the rectus abdominis laterally, flattening the lower abdomen.
- You should feel a deep, slow tensioning of the abdomen, not a fast bulging.

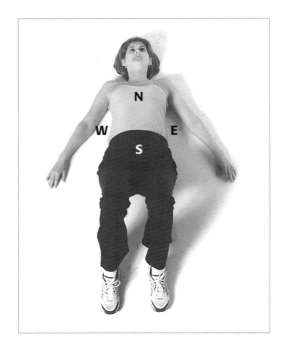

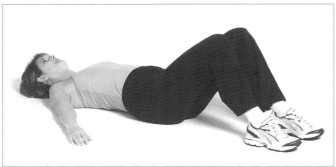

Fire the core and sustain lying supine.

Keep one finger on the TA and check the abdominals above your navel. These muscles should not be contracting; therefore, you should not feel your ribs moving. Do not hold your breath; concentrate on breathing normally.

Since expiration (breathing out) facilitates the action of the TA, breathing can be used as an assist or a challenge to this exercise. Moving with the breath has long been advocated by instructors of Pilates, yoga and Feldenkrais exercises. Take a small breath in and as you exhale, gently hollow the deep abdominals and draw the navel toward the spine.

Isolating the Multifidus

The multifidus is located deep within the lower back, right next to the bones in the midline of your spine and pelvis. It is contained within an envelope of fascia (connective tissue) which tightens when multifidus contracts. This increased fascial tension compresses the posterior pelvis and together with transversus abdominis completes the corset of the core.

Isolating Multifidus (sidelying)

• Lie on your side with your head supported on a pillow and your knees and hips bent.
• With one hand, palpate the multifidus muscle. You will find this muscle along both sides of the bony spine.
• Try to pull your hip up gently into its socket while feeling the muscle contract.

Progress to raising the top knee, keeping ankles together and maintaining the muscle contraction.

If you are unsure whether you are contracting the correct muscles, ask your healthcare

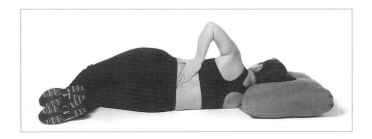

professional to assist you in isolating them. If you have had low back pain or sciatic symptoms it may be necessary to do extra "base work" exercises to ensure proper control of these muscles. See your physiotherapist for recommendations.

Exercises to Fire the Core and Sustain: Your Base Work

These exercises are not exhaustive and you may add others based on your experience or on the advice of your healthcare or fitness professional.

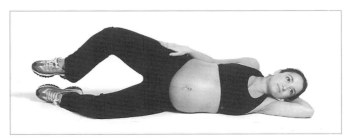

Isolating multifidus (sidelying).

Five on the Floor and More

These "Five on the Floor" exercises are ideal base work during the first trimester when it is safe to lie on your back for longer periods of time. As your pregnancy progresses past the first trimester, don't stay on your back more than 30 seconds or if you feel any discomfort or shortness of breath. During trimesters two and three these same exercises can be done sidelying or in an incline lying position.

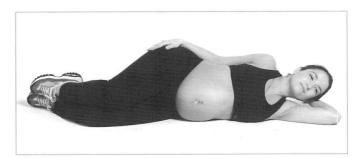

Sidelying position to exercise.

Fire the Core and Sustain

Before each exercise focus on the following:
• Contract the pelvic floor (Kegel).
• Contract the TA (lower abdominal).
• Remember to breathe.
• Keep knees soft if standing.

During each exercise follow these principles:
• Ensure that the initial contraction is isolated (no other muscles are substituting for the one to be worked).
• The contraction should begin slowly with control; very little effort is required.
• Breathe normally.

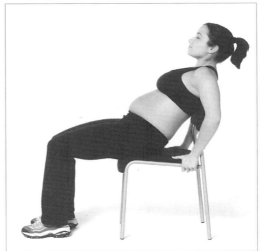

Incline lying position to exercise.

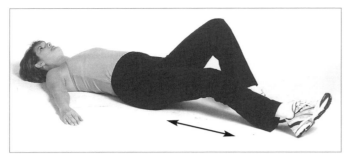

Supine leg slide.

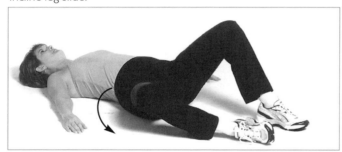

Incline leg slide.

1. Fire the Core and Sustain with Leg Slide

- Begin by lying on your back with your knees bent, and focus on isolating the TA with a normal breathing pattern.
- Keeping the TA contracted or "on" during the entire exercise, slowly straighten one leg while sliding it along the floor and then return to the start position, to a count of 10.
- Repeat with the other leg while you keep the TA "on" and continue to breathe.
- Repeat 10 times on each leg. This exercise can be made more challenging by lifting the foot off the floor as you slide it out and back.

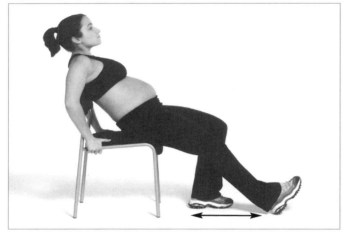

Supine leg fall out.

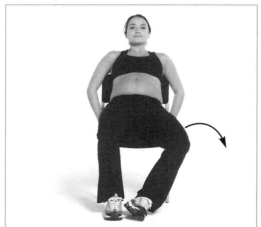

Incline leg fall out.

2. Fire the Core and Sustain with Leg Fall Out

- Find your TA while lying on your back, knees bent.
- Let one leg fall out to the side and raise it back up, to a count of 10.
- Don't let the opposite hip come up off the floor.
- Repeat 10 times on each leg.

3. Fire the Core and Sustain with March

- Find your TA while lying on your back, knees bent.
- March your feet up and down several inches to a count of 10.
- Don't raise your knees too high (not past 90 degrees).
- Repeat 10 times on each leg.

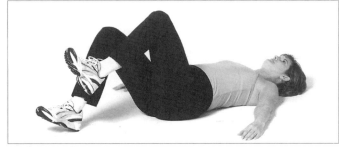
Supine march.

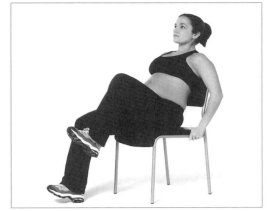
Incline march.

4. Fire the Core and Sustain with Limb Movement (Dying Bug)

- Find your TA while lying on your back, knees bent.
- Bring your opposite arm and knee to 90 degrees (they don't need to touch) and lower to a count of 10.
- Repeat 10 times on each side.

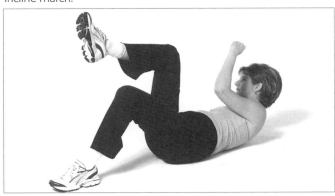
Supine dying bug.

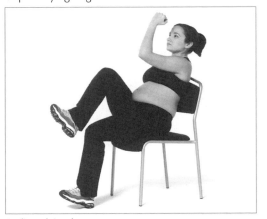
Incline dying bug.

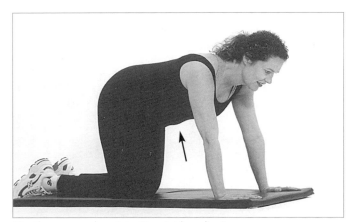

Fire the core and sustain (4-point kneeling).

5. Fire the Core and Sustain (4-Point Kneeling) (Pony Back–Neutral)

- Get down on all fours, ensuring that your shoulders and hips are centered over your hands and knees.
- Keep your low back in a neutral position (don't arch) and relax your abdomen.
- Take a breath in and then exhale, pulling your belly button up toward the spine.
- Hold this contraction of the TA for a count of 10, breathing normally.

Fire the Core and Sustain (Sitting)

- Sitting in a stable chair, find and maintain a neutral spine position.
- Take a normal breath in and as you exhale, slowly and gently draw your lower abdomen toward your spine.
- Feel the squeezing action produced by the co-activation of TA and multifidus.
- Challenge the TA activation by maintaining this deep contraction as you breathe in and out.
- Hold for 10 seconds, then relax and repeat. Aim to build up to 10 repetitions.

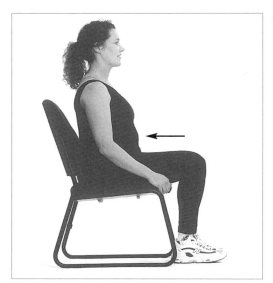

Fire the core and sustain (sitting).

Fire the Core and Sustain (Standing)

- Standing beside a mirror, find and maintain a neutral spine position.
- Take a normal breath in and as you exhale, slowly and gently draw your lower abdomen toward your spine.
- Feel the squeezing action produced by the co-activation of TA and multifidus. If you check in the mirror, you will see a slight indrawing of the lower abdomen.
- Challenge the core by maintaining this deep contraction as you breathe in and out.
- Hold for 10 seconds, then relax and repeat. Aim to build up to 10 repetitions.

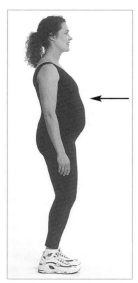

Fire the core and sustain (standing).

Fire the Core and Sustain (Weight Shifts)

- Stand beside a mirror, feet shoulder-width apart and knees slightly bent.
- Find and maintain a neutral spine position.
- Breathe in and as you exhale, draw your lower abdomen toward your spine.
- Once you feel the squeezing action of TA and multifidus, further challenge the core by shifting your weight forward and back, and side to side. Be careful not to let the knee go past the toe. You can increase the intensity by adding small hand weights.
- Hold for 10 seconds, then return to the starting position and repeat on the other leg. Aim to build up to 10 repetitions.

Fire the Core and Sustain (Sit to Stand A) (not shown)

- Sit on an exercise ball or chair with the spine in a neutral position.
- Breathe in and as you exhale, draw your lower abdomen toward your spine.
- Feel the squeezing action of TA and multifidus.
- Slowly stand up, keeping the core fired and making sure the knees don't go past the toes.

Fire the Core and Sustain (Sit to Stand B) (not shown)

- Sit on an exercise ball or chair with the spine in a neutral position.
- Breathe in and as you exhale, draw your lower abdomen toward your spine.
- Feel the squeezing action of TA and multifidus.
- Slowly stand up, keeping the core fired.
- Increase the intensity by holding a weight in each hand or stretching a piece of exer-

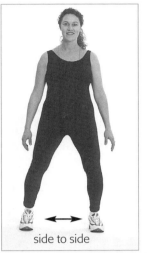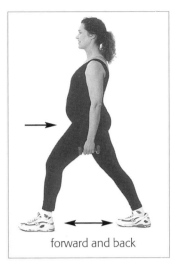

side to side | forward and back

Fire the core and sustain (weight shifts).

cise tubing in one hand or both as you stand.

Throughout the day, remember to fire the core and sustain prior to all activities that involve lifting, stepping, carrying, pushing or pulling.

Core Connections: Bringing it All Together

Stability and its Role in the Core

Stability is the capacity to control the amount of movement in your joints during loading, torsion and shear forces in multidirectional weight bearing. Each joint has a normal range of motion associated with it, and this range varies from person to person. Stability is how well you control the range of motion that you have, with specific individual muscles or groups of muscles.

During pregnancy and delivery, the muscles and joints of the lumbar spine (low back) and sacrum are weakened. This weakening is caused by a variety of different factors, including a change in circulating hormones. In addition, abdominal muscles are stretched by the growing fetus, and you may compensate for the extra weight up front by adjusting your posture—typically, with an arched back and slouched shoulders. The result can put a strain on the entire muscle and skeletal system, which can manifest itself with low back pain, neck strain and hip problems.

It becomes especially important during pregnancy to pay attention to the muscles of the abdominals and pelvic floor (PF-Core) because they are the most often stretched and weakened. Strengthening the PF-Core gives you a strong, stable base from which to work and move. If you don't have a strong base, certain parts of the body must absorb extra stress to compensate for the weak foundation.

The problems caused by this extra stress can continue long after childbirth unless the entire core, including the pelvic floor, is strengthened. Strengthening the entire muscle system helps alleviate pain and makes simple tasks—such as carrying a baby, getting in and out of the car, and lifting and reaching—much easier.

Now that you are able to properly fire the core and sustain it is time to connect the core to the extremities (arms and legs) with functional weight-bearing exercises.

The following exercises are designed to help develop the core and strengthen specific larger muscles in a dynamic and functional way. They are functional in nature and reflect the current research on how our muscles and fascial tissue link together to form sling systems connecting the core. These exercises are suitable for all fitness levels, and should be done before trying more advanced exercises. Before getting started perform the exercises outlined in chapter 5, Warm-up, and finish with cooldown exercises.

These exercises are not exhaustive and you may add others based on your experience or on the advice of your healthcare or fitness professional.

> **NOTE**
>
> *When adding other exercises to your fitness program, be sure to follow the ABCs of Smart Training (see chapter 4).*

First Trimester Only

Supine Bridging (stomach up)

- Lie on your back on a mat with your feet on the floor and knees bent to 90 degrees.
- Keep the head and arms relaxed.
- Your knees should be aligned directly over your toes and about hip-width apart.
- Fire the core and sustain; don't grip with your buttocks.
- Lift your hips and low back (from tailbone to ribcage) until trunk is level with thighs.
- Weight should be on the upper back, not the neck.
- Keep your spine neutral.
- Try it as well with knees and feet together for less stability.
- Hold for 4 seconds and do 2–3 sets of 10–15 repetitions.
- Strengthens core and hips.

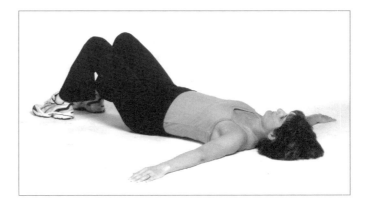

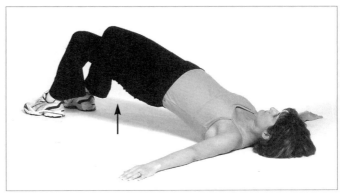

Supine bridging (stomach up).

Supine Bridging (with stretch cord abduction)

- Lie on your back on a mat with your feet on the floor and knees bent to 90 degrees.
- Keep the head and arms relaxed.
- Your knees should be aligned directly over your toes and about hip-width apart.
- Place a stretch cord around your knees.
- Fire the core and sustain, and push knees apart against stretch cord and lift your hips as above.
- Weight should be on the upper back, not the neck.
- Keep your spine neutral.
- Hold for 4 seconds and do 2–3 sets of 10–15 repetitions.
- Strengthens core and hips.

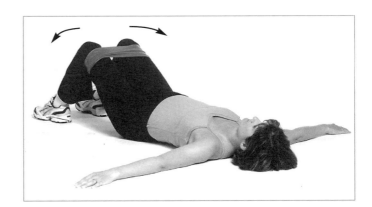

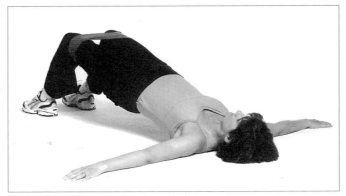

Supine bridging (with stretch cord abduction).

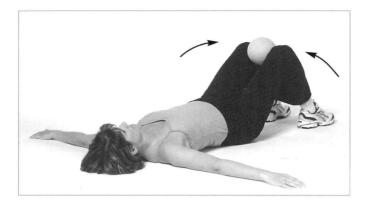

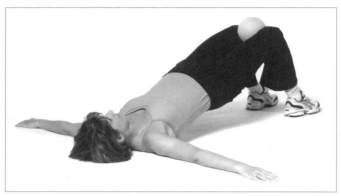

Supine bridging (with ball squeeze).

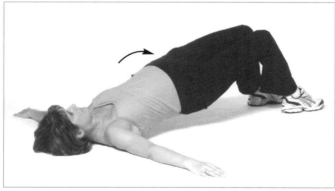

Bridge with rotation.

Supine Bridging (with ball squeeze)

- Lie on your back on a mat with your feet on the floor and knees bent to 90 degrees.
- Keep the head and arms relaxed.
- Your knees should be aligned directly over your toes and about hip-width apart.
- Place a small ball between your knees.
- Fire the core and sustain; don't grip with your buttocks.
- Squeeze the ball *very lightly* and bridge your hips up until your spine is neutral.
- Hold for 2–4 seconds and do 1–2 sets of 5–10 repetitions.
- Strengthens core and hips.

Caution: If you experience any groin pain discontinue this exercise.

Bridge with Rotation

- Lie on your back on a mat with your feet on the floor and knees bent to 90 degrees.
- Keep the head and arms relaxed.
- Your knees should be aligned directly over your toes and about hip-width apart.
- Fire the core and sustain; don't grip with your buttocks.
- Lift your hips and low back (from tail-bone to ribcage) until trunk is level with thighs.
- Weight should be on the upper back, not the neck.
- Keep your spine neutral and breathe normally.
- Breathe out and slowly rotate your pelvis to the right or left.
- Hold 4 seconds while breathing in, then breathe out to return to neutral.
- The movement is smooth and located in the hips; the knees remain still.
- Do 2–3 sets of 4 repetitions.
- Strengthens core and hips.

First, Second or Third Trimester
Clamshell

- Lie on your side with your head supported and your knees bent.
- Fire the core and sustain, keeping the contraction tight.
- Don't roll the pelvis and low back backward during this exercise.
- Slowly lift the top knee a few inches and then lower it back down. You should feel a compression force across the back of your pelvis.
- To make the exercise more difficult hold the top knee up and then slightly lift the top ankle. Slowly lower the ankle and then the knee.
- Do 2–3 sets of 10–15 repetitions.
- Strengthens core and lateral hip.

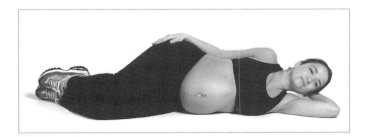

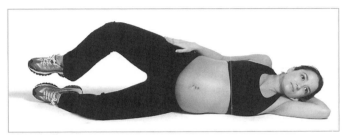

Clamshell.

Sidelying Leg Lifts

- Lie on your left side, left hand supporting your head, right hand on the floor in front of your tummy.
- Fire the core and sustain.
- Keep your hips forward, toes to the ceiling, and raise your leg up as far as your flexibility will allow, then return to starting position.
- Repeat on the other side.
- Do 2–3 sets of 10–15 repetitions.
- Strengthens core and lateral hip.

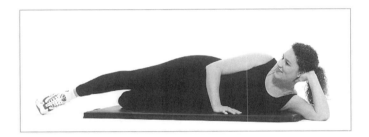

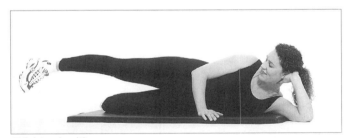

Sidelying leg lifts.

> **NOTE**
>
> *Supine bridging exercises that last more than 30 seconds can be done in the first trimester. During the second and third trimesters you can exercise for 30 seconds, then roll to your left side for a rest before continuing.*

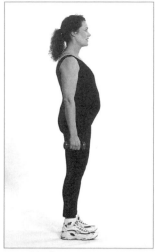
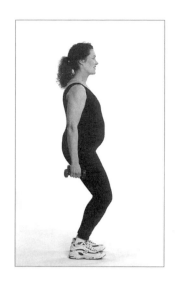

Dumbbell squats.

Dumbbell Squats

- Stand with your feet hip-width apart and your arms hanging at your sides, holding dumbbells.
- Keep your back straight and head up, and look straight ahead.
- Fire the core and sustain.
- Inhale as you squat until your thighs are parallel to the floor.
- While squeezing your glutes and pushing with your quadriceps, exhale as you return to the starting position.
- Do 2–3 sets of 10–15 repetitions.
- Strengthens core and front thighs.

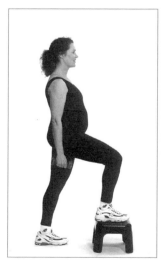
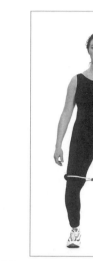

Squats with stretch cord resistance.

Squats with Stretch Cord Resistance

- Stand tall, and fire the core and sustain.
- Place a stretch cord around your legs, just above your knees.
- With hips square, push the stretch cord out lightly as you squat.
- Can be done with weights or with hands on hips.
- Do 2–3 sets of 10–15 repetitions.
- Strengthens core, front and lateral thighs.

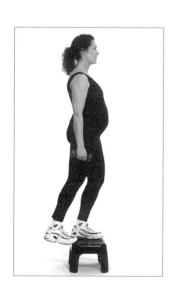

Front step-ups.

Front Step-ups

- Stand facing a low stool or step, and fire the core and sustain while keeping your shoulders back.
- Holding a dumbbell in each hand, exhale as you step up onto the stool.
- This exercise can be done with or without weights.
- Ensure that the stool you are stepping onto is not placing your knee beyond 90 degrees.
- Do 2–3 sets of 10–15 repetitions.
- Strengthens core and front thighs.

Side Step-ups

- Stand beside a low (approximately 4–6 inches high) bench, and fire the core and sustain while keeping your shoulders back.
- Holding a dumbbell in each hand, exhale as you step up sideways onto the bench.
- This exercise can be done with or without weights.
- Do 2–3 sets of 10–15 repetitions.
- Strengthens front and lateral thighs.

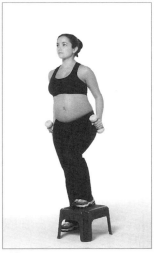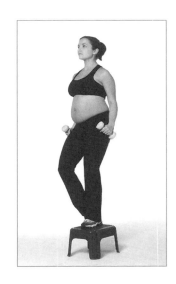

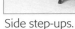
Side step-ups.

Alternating Standing Lunges

- Stand with your feet together and arms at your sides.
- Fire the core and sustain.
- Keeping your back straight and your head up, take a large step forward.
- Bend until your front thigh is parallel to the floor, ensuring that at the bottom of the movement your front knee does not pass your toes. Your back leg should be almost straight and should not touch the floor.
- Always exhale on exertion.
- This exercise can be done with or without weights.
- Do 2–3 sets of 10–15 repetitions.
- Strengthens thighs and buttocks.

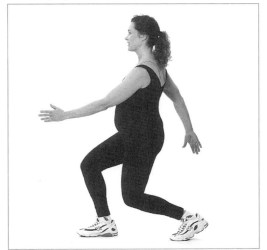
Alternate standing lunges.

Circus Ponies (alternating arm and leg raise)

- Start on your hands and knees.
- Keep your back in a neutral position, and fire the core and sustain.
- Exhale as you raise the opposite arm and leg.
- Hold this position for 4 seconds.
- Do 2–3 sets of 10–15 repetitions.
- Strengthens core and lower back.

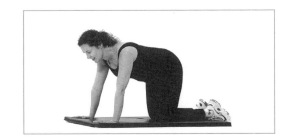

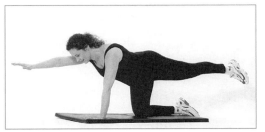
Circus ponies.

Kegel Exercises for a Strong Pelvic Floor

Performing Kegel exercises is very important for both pregnant and postpartum women. Kegel exercises are done by contracting the pelvic floor muscles in a regular and controlled fashion. Although comparable to stopping and starting the flow of urine, these exercises actually contract and lift the delivery canal. This ensures healthy vaginal tissue and assists with urinary control while pregnant, during delivery and postpartum.

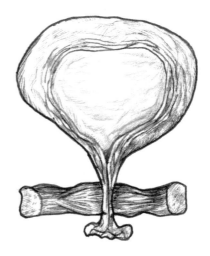

Bladder, urethra and pelvic floor muscles.

> **NOTE**
>
> *Never practice Kegels while urinating as this may increase your chance of getting a bladder infection.*

The Kegel contraction can be analyzed in three parts: the urethral, vaginal and anal contraction. It is difficult to separate these three because we are not accustomed to performing these exercises. Also, these muscles work more in tandem than separately. When performing a Kegel, the vaginal canal is contracted along with the entire pelvic floor, and therefore the anal area also experiences a contraction. A repeated contraction and release in the anal area may help prevent hemorrhoids because the muscles stimulate the veins and increase circulation. This increases peripheral blood flow or venous return, making it less likely that blood will pool and veins will expand. (Kegels will not prevent hemorrhoids completely as genetics are the greatest factor in determining whether or not you will get varicose veins, including hemorrhoids, during pregnancy.)

Practicing the release of the Kegel may also assist with the function of the large intestine and with defecation. This may help to prevent the constipation that can plague many pregnant women.

While practicing Kegel exercises, it is as important to perform the release or relaxation phase as it is to perform the muscle contraction. When you experience your first contraction—which can be somewhat scary for first-time mothers—your initial reaction

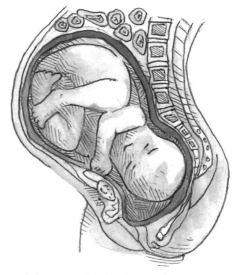

Abdomen and pelvic floor in third trimester.

may be to contract the entire pelvic floor. This full-body tensing reaction is much like the way in which you slam on the brakes to stop your car in an accident situation. However, you must learn to relax your pelvic floor during a contraction. Contractions in labor are a tightening of the uterus that may cause a general contraction of the entire abdominal region. The contracting uterus helps to push the baby down in the final phase of labor, but if the pelvic floor is tightened this may hinder the progression of labor.

You should incorporate the following exercises into your cooldown routine to ensure they are not forgotten. Sitting on an exercise ball, Sissel disc, foam roll or rolled towel will give you an unstable base of support and make the exercises more challenging. Remember that the quality of these exercises, not the quantity, is most important.

The nice thing about Kegels is that nobody knows you are exercising! It's easy to fit in these exercises while you are:

- Waiting for a bus
- Ironing or cooking
- Watching TV
- Standing in line
- Having sex
- Stopped at a red light
- Cuddling your baby
- Sitting in a meeting or waiting room.

Slow Hold (Hold-ems)

- Sit or lie comfortably with your legs wide apart.
- Close your eyes and imagine that you want to "hold on" and stop yourself from passing urine or wind.

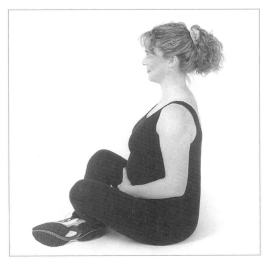
Floor Kegels.

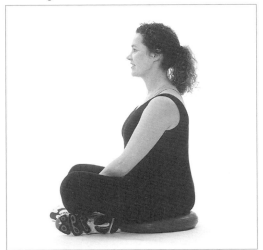
Sissel disc Kegels.

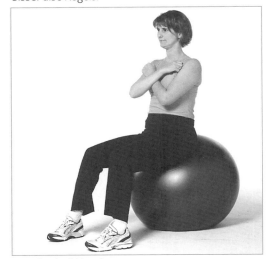
Exercise ball Kegels.

- Squeeze the muscles around your front passage (vagina) and back passage (anus) as strongly as possible and hold tightly for 3 seconds. By doing this you should feel the pelvic floor muscles lift up inside. Relax for at least 5 seconds.
- Repeat this "squeeze and lift" movement up to 10 times, holding the contraction for 3–5 seconds or as long as 10–15 seconds if you are able. Ensure that the squeeze stays strong and you can feel the "let go."
- Rest for 1 minute before you proceed to the next exercise.

Quick Squeeze (Speed-ems)

- Squeeze and lift the pelvic floor muscles as strongly and quickly as possible. Don't try to hold on to the contraction; just squeeze and let go.
- Gradually increase the speed of each contraction and the number of repetitions before the muscle tires. Allow a 3-second rest in between each exercise.
- Repeat 10 times. Do this several times a day.

Squeeze and Hold (Squeeze-ems)

- Squeeze the pelvic floor muscles and hold for a slow count of 5 to start, working your way up to 10. Relax and rest for 10 seconds.
- Repeat 5–10 times. Do this several times a day.

Elevator Exercise (Elevate-ems)

- Visualize your midsection as an apartment tower. Using your pelvic floor muscles, draw upwards to the first floor and hold for 5 seconds.

- While continuing to hold, draw upwards to the second floor and hold for 5 seconds.
- Release and repeat several times per day. Sitting on a pillow, ball or Sissel disc will help increase your ability to contract.

Belly Button Breathing

- Using your diaphragm draw a breath in through your nose.
- Exhale through your mouth as you say HA HA HA.
- Do 1–3 sets of 10 repetitions.

Baby Hugs

- Sitting with your back supported, use your transverse abdominals to wrap around your baby or a pillow and give it a hug.
- Give your baby or pillow a bigger hug, then the biggest hug. Your belly button should be pulling toward the spine.
- Do 1–3 sets of 10 repetitions.

During the above exercises you should not:
- feel any downward movement as you contract the muscles
- tighten your thighs or buttocks
- hold your breath.

In addition to these specific exercises, remember to tense up your pelvic floor every time you cough, sneeze or lift—most people do this automatically. Regular general exercise will also have a positive effect on the strength of your pelvic floor muscles. Once you feel confident about doing these exercises you may try them in different positions such as standing, or lying on your back, side or stomach.

To prevent further damage to pelvic floor muscles, avoid:

• constipation and/or straining with a bowel movement
• persistent heavy lifting
• repetitive coughing or sneezing.

For many women it is important to follow a specific exercise program tailored to their individual needs. If you are unsure whether you are exercising these muscles correctly, or if you have urinary problems, you should consult your physician and see a women's health physical therapist.

Diastasis in Abdominal Muscles

The abdominal muscles form a strong but elastic "wall" behind which your baby can grow safely in the uterus. The abdominals also help to support your spine and assist in good posture. In about 30% of pregnant women the central muscles of the abdomen (the rectus abdominis muscle) will separate due to the increasing tension of the growing baby. This is called diastasis recti abdominis, and it needs to be minimized or corrected to allow the abdominal muscles to function properly.

Self Test for Diastasis Recti Abdominis

Lying flat on your back with your knees bent, place your little finger in the navel between the two rectus muscles and your three other fingers in a straight line toward your breastbone. Slowly lift your head until your shoulders come off the floor and turn your fingers 90 degrees to check how many fingers can be inserted between the two muscles. If the separation is three or more fingers you should do the corrective exercise

below and avoid traditional sit-ups, which can exacerbate the problem. You may want to speak to your caregiver for clarification.

Corrective Exercise for Diastasis Recti

Though on first glance this appears to be a traditional sit-up, your hand placement assists the split rectus muscle. Lie flat on your back with your knees bent and your hands folded over your abdomen so that they support the abdominal muscles. Inhale, and while slowly exhaling, raise your head to your chest. Hold this position for two normal breaths, then gently lower your head to the floor. Repeat this exercise 10 times. In your second and third trimester, use an incline bench.

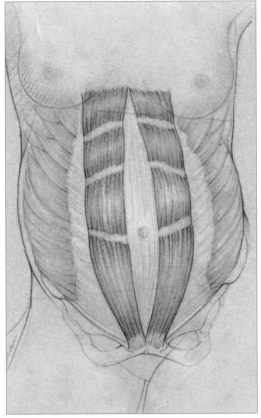

Diastasis recti abdominis.

Postural Changes and Exercises

The physical changes in your body during pregnancy lead to changes in posture. The most common change is the pelvis tilting forward (anteriorly) on one or both sides. The lower back (lumbar) curve is increased, the knees tend to straighten (hyperextend), the shoulders slouch and the head is carried forward. As well, the ribs flare out in an effort to allow you to take deeper breaths. These changes result from a forward shift in your center of gravity as the baby grows and the breasts enlarge.

The hormone relaxin causes the joints, particularly in the pelvis, to become more lax to help prepare the body for birth and to allow your baby to pass more easily through the birth canal. The increase in relaxin changes your hormonal balance and can contribute to malalignment of the low back and pelvis, which may lead to low back pain or problems with the weight-bearing joints. This joint laxity can also cause a flare-up of old injuries as you find yourself walking with a wider base of support—the typical pregnant "waddle"—to compensate for the increased weight and redistribution of body mass. Everyday activities such as walking, stooping, stair climbing, lifting and reaching may become difficult. The upward shift in your center of balance can also put you at a higher risk of falling when exercising, and you should keep this in mind as your pregnancy progresses. Ensure that you include some balance training exercises in your fitness program (see chapter 8 for ideas).

Improving Your Posture

Maintaining good posture throughout the day can help to relieve some of the discomforts associated with pregnancy. Good body alignment involves utilizing the muscles closest to the spine. Picture each segment of the spine as a building block. If alignment is correct the blocks stack evenly on one another. However, if any are out of alignment some external forces (the interspinal muscles) must be used to hold them up, and the constant tension required in the muscles to keep your spine upright can lead to muscle fatigue and pain.

Regular exercise can help offset the effects of pregnancy on ligamentous laxity by improving the joint sense (proprioception) and improving strength and muscle tone around the joint. Targeted strength and core exercises may help reduce the incidence of low back pain and other common muscle and joint complaints. These exercises will also minimize the inevitable upward and outward shift in your center of gravity as your uterus grows and protrudes, by maintaining back strength and strong abdominal muscle tone.

> **NOTE**
>
> *Prolonged pressure on the spinal joints and discs from poor posture and sitting habits can cause irritation and eventual damage. If you will be sitting in one place for any length of time (for example, while watching TV, listening to music or reading), to decrease spinal pressure it is best to lie with your feet up or in a semi-reclining position.*

Proper Standing Posture

- Feet shoulder-width apart and parallel
- Weight evenly distributed
- Knees soft (slightly bent)
- Tension in buttocks and lower abdominals
- Tummy tight
- Shoulder blades squeezed together
- Shoulders relaxed and down
- Chin in
- Eyes level

Proper Seated Posture

- Buttocks to back of chair
- Pelvis vertical
- Shoulders above hips
- Tension in buttocks and lower abdominals
- Tummy tight
- Shoulder blades squeezed together
- Shoulders relaxed and down
- Chin in
- Eyes level

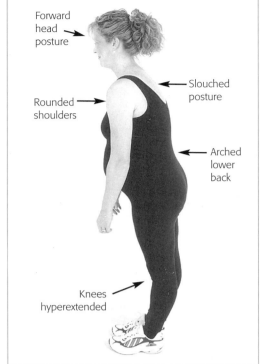
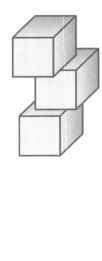

Forward head posture

Slouched posture

Rounded shoulders

Arched lower back

Knees hyperextended

Poor posture.

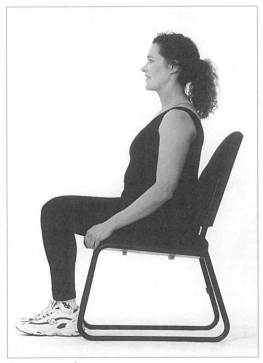

Proper seated posture.

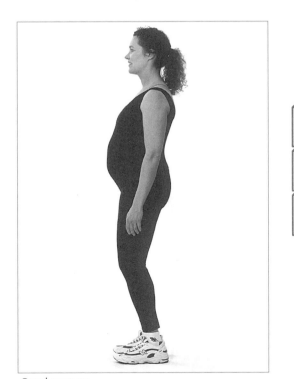

Good posture.

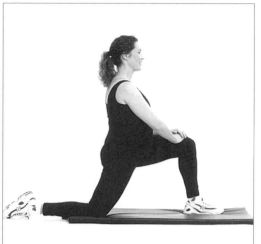

Hip flexor stretch (kneeling).

The following stretches and strength exercises will help improve posture.

Stretch the muscles that tend to be short and stiff:

Hip Flexor Stretch (kneeling)

- Kneel on the floor with one leg forward.
- Press your back hip forward, feeling the stretch at the front of the thigh.
- Hold for 20–40 seconds and repeat 2–3 times.

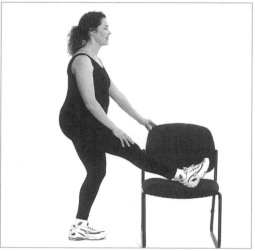

Hamstring stretch.

Hamstring Stretch

- Stand in front of a low table or chair and place one straight leg on top, keeping hips square.
- Lean from waist, keeping chest up, and exhale as you bend forward.
- Hold for 20–40 seconds and repeat 2–3 times each side.

TIPS FROM THE TEAM

- Stretch out the muscles that may tend to be stiff, like the hip flexors, quadriceps, hamstrings, lower back and pectorals (chest).
- Strengthen the muscles that tend to get weak, like the abdominals, gluteals (buttocks), hamstrings and upper back.

- Pay attention to your balance. Use a wall or chair to stabilize yourself while stretching.
- A health and fitness professional can advise you on correct lifting and carrying techniques.

Pectoral Stretch

- Place one arm on the wall with elbow bent at 90 degrees and below shoulder height.
- Push shoulder forward until you feel a stretch in the chest.
- Hold for 10–15 seconds and repeat 2–3 times each side.

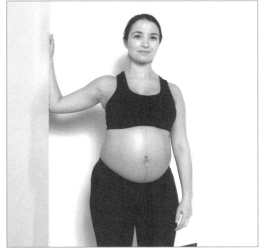

Pectoral stretch.

Strengthen muscles that are usually long and weak:

Fire the Core and Sustain with March

- Fire the core and sustain while lying on your back, knees bent.
- March your feet up and down several inches for a count of 10 seconds.
- Don't raise your knees too high (not past 90 degrees).
- Repeat 10 times.

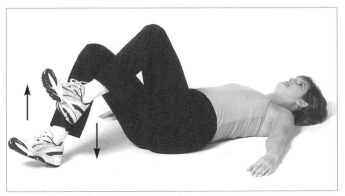

Fire the core and sustain with march.

Shoulder Blade Retractions with Stretch Cord

- Fire the core and sustain while standing with knees slightly bent.
- Pull a stretch cord to your chest and then pull apart.
- Do 10–15 repetitions and repeat 2–3 times.

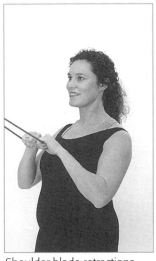
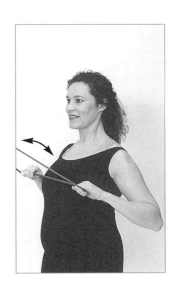

Shoulder blade retractions.

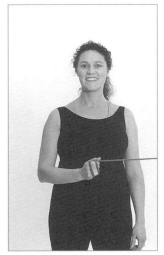 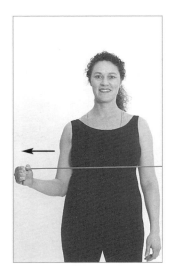

Posterior shoulder.

Posterior Shoulder (Infraspinatus) with Stretch Cord

- Fire the core and sustain while standing with knees slightly bent.
- Keep your elbow at your side throughout the exercise.
- Holding a stretch cord, exhale as you rotate your arm away from your body.
- Do 10–15 repetitions and repeat 2–3 times.

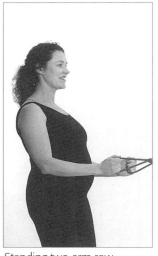 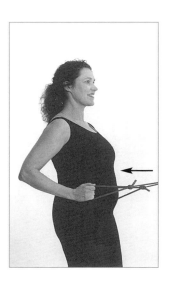

Standing two-arm row.

Standing Two-Arm Row

- Fire the core and sustain while standing with knees slightly bent and shoulders square.
- Keeping your shoulders down, exhale as you bring your elbows back until wrists meet hips.
- Do 10–15 repetitions and repeat 2–3 times.

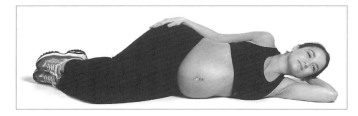

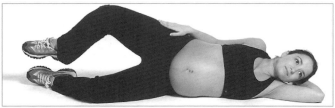

Clamshell.

Hip Lateral Rotators (Gluteals)

- Lying on your side, fire the core and sustain.
- Raise upper knee about 8 to 10 inches, like opening up a clamshell.
- Hold for 2–4 seconds and lower.
- Do 10–15 repetitions and repeat 2–3 times.

Carrying and Lifting During Pregnancy and Postpartum

Proper Posture

All of the exercises in this book help prepare you to care for your newborn, but ensuring proper posture while carrying and lifting your infant is the best way to prevent discomfort and injury.

> *Focus on proper lifting technique when you lift anything.*

Proper Lifting Technique

- Always fire the core and sustain before you begin.
- Keep the load close to the body. Avoid moving it outside your base of support.
- Check that the load is not too heavy before lifting it, and get help if necessary.

Always protect your back when lifting your infant. For example, if the crib side rails drop only halfway down and you must lean over them to reach your baby, make sure you stand with your feet well apart to give you a better base of support for lifting. Contract your core and think about lifting in one fluid motion. You will have fewer hand and wrist problems if you lift your baby from his or her base—one hand behind the neck and the other hand under the buttocks—because in this position, postural reflexes keep the baby upright and make him or her easier for you to hold.

When lifting your infant out of the back seat of a two-door car or the center seat of a four-door car, climb in and sit beside the infant seat. Lift your baby onto your lap and emerge as a unit, supporting from his or her base. If your child is on either the passenger's or driver's side, be sure to bend your knees and contract your TA and Kegel when you lift your child into and out of the car. Pull the child close to your chest and emerge from the car as one unit.

Changing Positions During Pregnancy

Before pregnancy you likely didn't give much thought to getting out of bed or sitting up. But now with the extra load and changes to your center of gravity, you need to pay more attention to position changes to avoid excess stress on the muscles and joints.

Getting down to the floor

To get down to the floor without putting your back and neck at risk: Gently lower yourself down on one knee, keeping your back as straight as possible, then bring your other knee down. Take your hands to one side and rest them on the floor, so that they

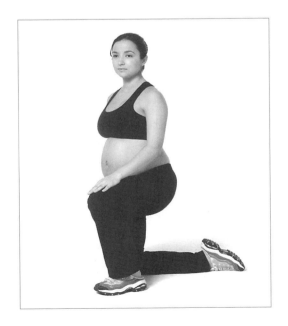

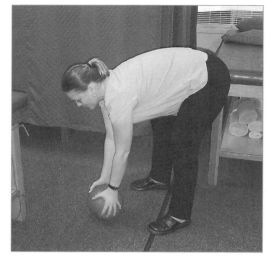

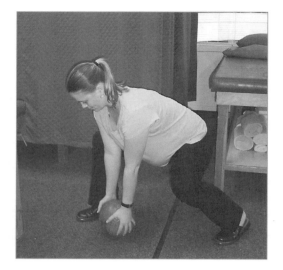

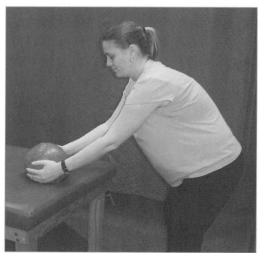

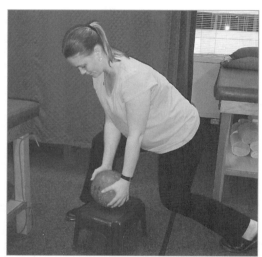

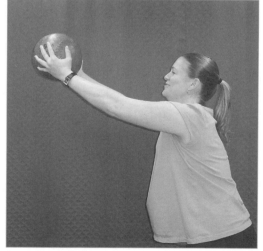

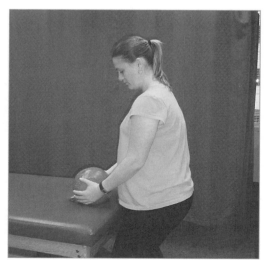

Improper techniques.

Proper techniques.

can support your weight as you shift your hips to one side. Ease your legs out to the side and lower yourself slowly to the floor.

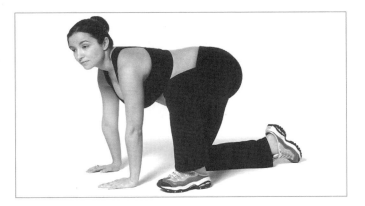

Getting up from the floor

Do the reverse of above: Lie on your side and then lift your upper body so that you are kneeling, and bring one leg up in front of you. Put your hands on your upper thigh and use the muscles in your legs to help you up from the floor.

Sitting to standing

Put your hands above your knees, take a belly breath, fire the core and sustain the transverse abdominals, lean forward and use your arms to push yourself up.

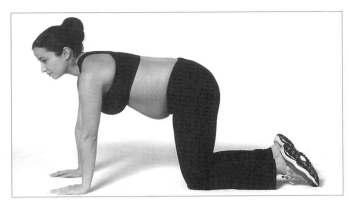

Sitting to lying on your back

Roll onto one hip and use your arms to ease yourself down, then roll onto your back.

Lying on your back to sitting

Roll to one side, keeping head neutral. Push yourself up with your hands, maintaining a neutral spine and letting your head come up last.

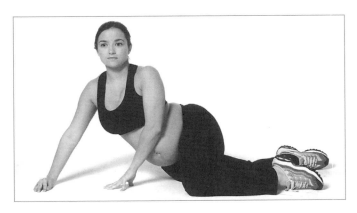

Getting out of the car

Move both legs and knees as a unit and let your torso follow in alignment, to avoid any torsion to the spine. Use the door and steering wheel for assistance standing up.

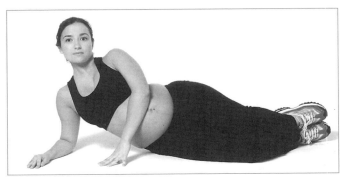

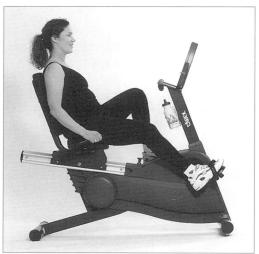

Aerobic Training

Various aerobic activities are used in conjunction with the strengthening aspects of the Fit to Deliver program to boost the aerobic benefit. Research suggests that doing aerobic activity has the greatest impact on the prevention of diseases and on maternal well-being during pregnancy (Clapp, 1994).

Alignment

It is important to maintain correct anatomical alignment to allow for proper force distribution upon your body's weight-bearing

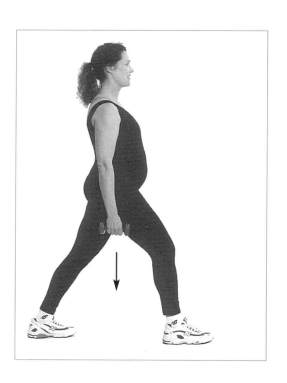

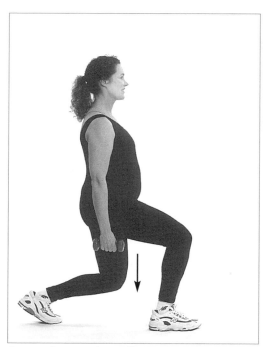

Proper alignment in a split squat.

structures during activity. Start with excellent alignment of the spine—imagine someone pulling you up by the top of your head, lengthening your spine. The neck should be long and the shoulders relaxed and down. Emphasize correct knee alignment, with knees always tracking over the toes but not going past them. When doing lunges or split squats ensure the line of gravity is through the pubic bone (center of the body), to avoid shear forces on the pelvis. If you are unsure about your posture or alignment consult with your fitness professional or physical therapist.

- Stand tall and practice good posture.
- Knees track in line with the toes.
- Line of gravity through pubic symphysis.

Balance Exercises

Good balance is fundamental for mobility and dynamic activity. Balance exercises should be included as a component of every fitness program. Working on balance is even more important now as the hormone relaxin decreases the ligament stability you need to improve muscle strength and balance control. You want to continually reset your balance clock and give your body the opportunity to practice moving with your newly changed muscles and altered joint stability (see chapter 8 for more information on balance training).

Balanced Body Strengthening and Stretching

Balanced training ensures that equal stress is put on the different parts of the body. Strength training should include exercises for all of the following areas:

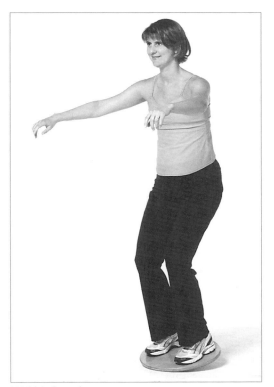

Wobble board.

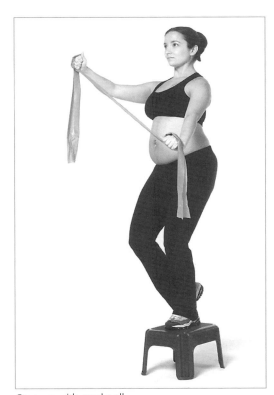

Step-up with cord pull.

- right and left sides
- flexor and extensor muscles
- medial and lateral rotator muscles
- upper and lower body and core. Try three or four each of upper body, lower body and core exercises to ensure a good balance (see chapter 7, Strength or Resistance Training).

Include stretches for both the front and back of the arms, legs and torso (see Smart Stretching Guidelines in chapter 5).

Consistency

Strive to train for a minimum of 4 to 6 days per week to provide maximum benefits to you and your baby.

Core and Pelvic Floor

The core and pelvic floor muscles should be fired and sustained during all exercise and daily activity. Aim to develop a strong, stable platform for your extremities (arms and legs) to work off. Pelvic floor exercises (Kegels) should also be practiced often throughout pregnancy (see chapter 3, The Core).

Diversity in Training

Use a variety of different training methods in your program to avoid boredom and overload. For example, core training may use a mix of floor, standing, ball and stretch cord exercises. Diversify training by altering exercises, altering the sequence of exercises and changing the tempo.

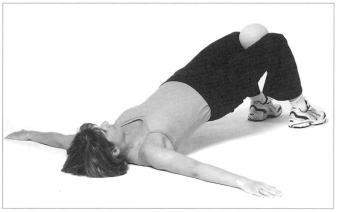

Core exercise—supine bridge and ball squeeze.

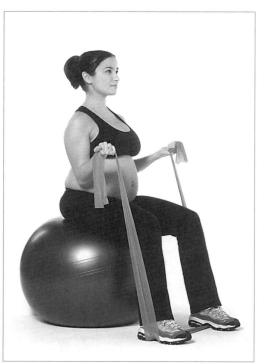

Bicep curls on exercise ball.

Dynamic Exercises

Your training should include exercises that promote dynamic flexibility and strength. This type of exercise improves general fitness but also helps you in your normal activities of daily living, like lifting, stepping, carrying, pushing or pulling. Choose exercises that focus on connecting the core to activity and that combine upper body, lower body and core movements.

Exercise at a Slow and Controlled Tempo

Each repetition should take 3 to 4 seconds to complete. This will help build endurance and strength without putting too much stress on the soft tissues. Never use momentum to perform an exercise or do exercises that are uncontrolled. Put extra emphasis on the lengthening (eccentric) portion of the exercise.

Fun

Choose exercises that you really enjoy. Your workout should be fun and leave you feeling invigorated, both mentally and physically.

Functional and Good Form

Do functional exercises that mimic your everyday activities. Practice correct form and correct breathing (no breath holding), and always fire the core and sustain during any exercise.

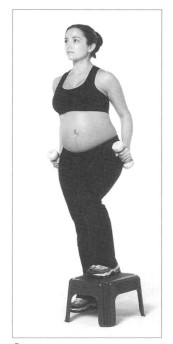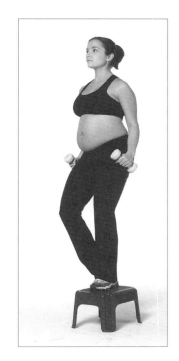

Step ups.

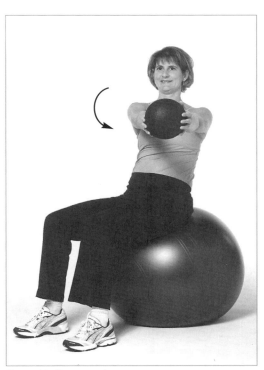

Seated ball torso twists.

Warm-up

The warm-up is an important component to training. It consists of a group of exercises performed immediately before an activity and provides a period of adjustment from rest to exercise. Experts agree that a warm-up prior to any activity, including stretching, is advisable. Warming up the body slowly helps prevent injuries caused by going too hard, too fast with cold, unlubricated muscles and joints. A good way to warm up is to

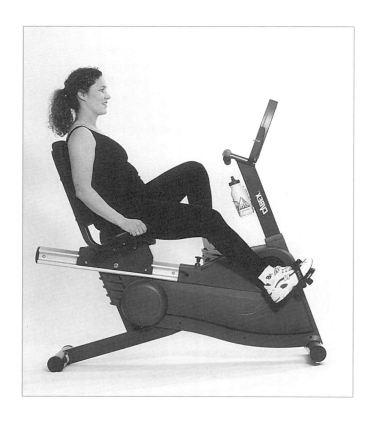

perform a less intense version of the activity you are doing. For example, if you are running, start off at half speed, then follow with some light static stretching. The Fit to Deliver program takes basic warm-ups one step further to include dynamic warm-ups.

The Fit to Deliver Dynamic Warm-up

A *dynamic warm-up* incorporates stretching exercises that prepare the muscles and joints in different planes of motion for the upcoming activity and serve to switch on the nervous system. Examples of dynamic stretches include crossovers, side shuffles, high knees and heel drills or skips. Using this type of stretching in a warm-up helps normalize joint mechanics and movement patterns, increase dynamic range of motion of the joints and decrease compensatory hypermobility (increased movement) in other areas. As well, dynamic stretching helps improve balance to the joints and improves relaxation and contraction coordination of the muscles. Always *begin dynamic stretching* with small muscles and small movements in a controlled range and *end dynamic stretching* with larger muscles in larger and more dynamic movements.

A dynamic warm-up optimally prepares your body for the demands of exercise. It should be performed before each exercise session, and should last 7 to 10 minutes and focus on the major muscle groups of the body. Note: Warm-ups take longer in cold temperatures and in pregnant women. Begin with a low level cardiovascular activity (traditional warm-up), then follow with dynamic stretching (exercises listed below) and static stretching. When you have broken a light sweat you are sufficiently warmed up.

> **NOTE**
>
> *You should do a specific warm-up before every training session to prepare yourself mentally as well as physically.*

Dynamic Warm-up and Cooldown

These exercises are not exhaustive and you may add others based on your experience or on the advice of your healthcare or fitness professional.

Always Fire the Core and Sustain

Before each exercise focus on the following:
• Contract the pelvic floor (Kegel).
• Contract the TA (lower abdominal).
• Remember to breathe.
• Keep knees soft (slightly bent) if standing.

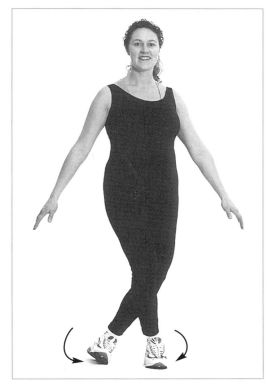

Crossovers.

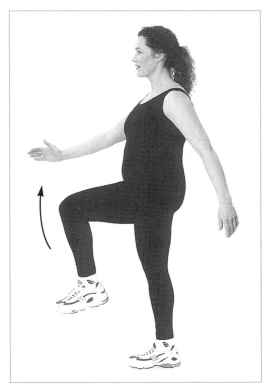

High knees march.

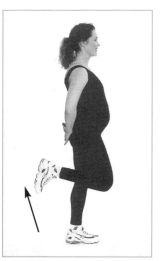

Butt kicks.

Butt Kicks

- Stand tall, and fire the core and sustain to make sure your hips are square.
- Bring your heel to your butt, alternating legs.
- Do 2 sets of 5–10 repetitions.

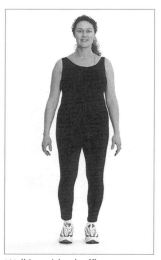 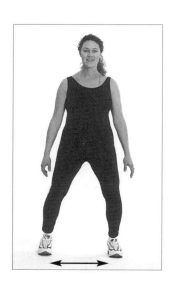

Walking side shuffles.

Walking Side Shuffles

- Stand with your feet shoulder-width apart, and fire the core and sustain. Take a wide step to the right and then step together with your left foot.
- Do 2 sets of 5–10 repetitions in each direction.

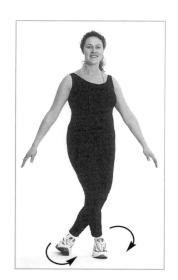

Walking crossovers.

Walking Crossovers

- Stand with your core fired and hips square. Walking sideways, cross your right foot behind your left leg and step left with your left foot, then cross your right foot in front and step left again.
- Do 2 sets of 5–10 steps in each direction.

High Knees

- Stand with your core fired, hips and shoulders square. Lift one knee up to 90 degrees, alternating right and left legs.
- Do 2 sets of 5–10 repetitions with each leg.

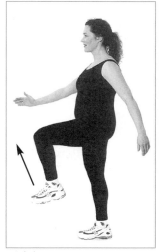

High knees.

Leg Swings (front and back)

- Holding onto a chair for support with your hips square, gently swing your leg forward and back. Remember to keep your supporting knee slightly bent, and fire the core and sustain.
- Do 2 sets of 5–10 repetitions.

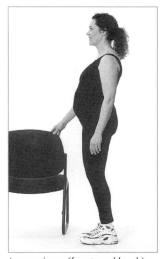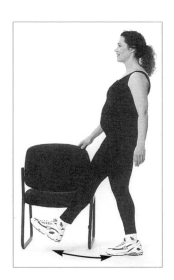

Leg swings (front and back).

Leg Swings (side to side)

- Bring your leg in front of your body and swing it gently from side to side, keeping your core fired, knees slightly bent and standing tall.
- Do 2 sets of 5–10 repetitions.

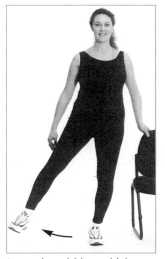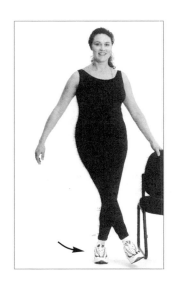

Leg swings (side to side).

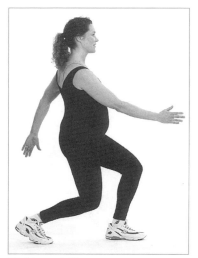

Walking mini lunges.

Walking Mini Lunges

- Stand tall with your shoulders back, and keep your core fired and sustain. Take a small step forward and lower your back knee toward the floor but do not allow it to touch. Your front knee should bend to about 60 degrees.
- Do 2 sets of 5–10 repetitions on each leg.

Torso Twists

- Stand with knees soft (slightly bent), and fire the core and sustain. Place hands on hips and slowly rotate your torso to the side up to 45 degrees.
- Hold for 10–15 seconds and repeat 2–3 times on each side.

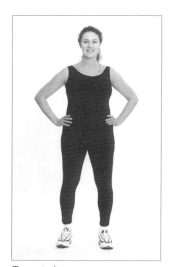
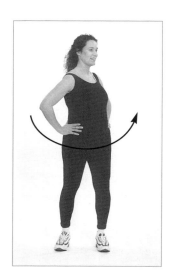

Torso twists.

Ankle Rotations (not shown)

- Lift one leg off the ground. Gently draw a small circle with the foot, clockwise and then counter-clockwise.
- Do 5–10 repetitions in each direction.

Shoulder Rolls (not shown)

- Stand with feet shoulder-width apart and knees soft.
- Roll shoulders forward and back.
- Try doing 5–10 repetitions in each direction.

Arm Swings

- Stand with feet shoulder-width apart and knees soft, keeping the core fired and sustain.
- Try swinging arms front to back, side to side and in a figure-8 motion.
- Start slowly and gradually increase the range of motion.

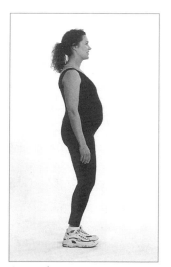
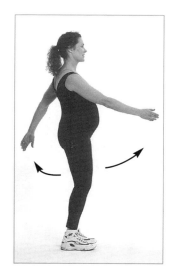

Arm swings.

Wrist Rotations (not shown)

- Gently roll wrists clockwise, then counter-clockwise.
- Try doing 5–10 repetitions in each direction.

Cooldown

A cooldown gradually takes your body back to its resting state, bringing down the heart rate and body temperature. During exercise, skeletal muscle contraction helps the venous system return blood to the heart. If exercise is stopped abruptly, blood will pool at the feet and leave the exerciser feeling lightheaded. This is especially dangerous in pregnant women because of increased blood volume and increased vasodilatation. Cooling down also helps prevent delayed onset muscle soreness and residual muscle tension by aiding in the removal of waste products from the muscle.

For an adequate cooldown try 8–10 minutes of moderate to light activity that is rhythmical in nature, followed by an easy general static stretch. Be sure to stretch all muscle groups used in the activity. Take care to stretch only to the point of tension, not pain, and hold each stretch for at least 30–40 seconds. Always perform some core strength and Kegel exercises at the end of your exercise program. Incorporating some balance training exercises is also recommended.

Smart Stretching Guidelines

When time is at a premium, often the first component of our exercise program to be neglected is the most boring part: stretching. But stretching is especially important to your overall physical health during pregnancy, not only to aid recovery and keep the body moving well but also to prevent injury.

TIPS FROM THE TEAM

1. Dynamic stretches move the joints through range of motion as part of a specific warm-up.

2. Allow a minimum of 10 to 15 minutes for stretching; a more comprehensive session may take 30 to 40 minutes.

3. Do 1 or 2 sets of 5 to 10 repetitions.

4. If a particular stretch causes discomfort, try an alternative. Stretching should NEVER be painful.

5. Include one stretch for each major muscle group.

6. If a particular muscle group is stiff stretch it first and last.

7. If the muscle is contracting to support your weight it cannot lengthen; therefore all exercises that are designed to lengthen muscles should be done passively in a relaxed manner.

8. Stay within your normal range of motion when doing dynamic warm-up. Don't over-stretch.

9. When doing these stretches do not use any resistance.

10. Ankles, legs and hands often swell during pregnancy. Try elevating feet and pumping ankles to reduce the swelling.

11. Watch yourself in a mirror to ensure proper form and alignment.

Due to an increase in weight and a shift in your center of gravity certain muscles—the hamstrings, low back extensors, pectorals, hip flexors and gluteals—tend to shorten. When these muscles are short and stiff they are less able to absorb shock and this can lead to stress on other areas. Stretching these muscles to ensure their optimal length, and to restore balance, can help to minimize some common pregnancy discomforts such as low back pain.

You should do dynamic and static stretching daily after a proper warm-up (you have broken a light sweat) and during the cooldown period. If you're running late, stretch at home while on the phone or watching television. The benefits of both types of stretching include:

- Improvement or maintenance of range of motion
- Reduction of injuries caused by tearing of tight soft tissue
- Promotion of muscle relaxation
- Increased metabolism in muscles, joints and associated connective tissue
- Enhanced physical fitness and improved body awareness
- Reduction in problems associated with delayed onset muscle soreness.

> **NOTE**
> *It is better to do many short stretches throughout the day than to do none at all.*

Caution: During pregnancy the hormone relaxin affects most joints of the body, making overstretching a possibility. Be very careful not to exceed your normal range of motion.

Relaxin is still present in your body up to four months postpartum (longer if you are breastfeeding), and therefore you should closely monitor your stretching during the postpartum period as well.

Different Types of Stretching
Dynamic Stretching

Dynamic stretching used as a warm-up helps normalize joint mechanics, increases the dynamic range of motion, improves joint position sensors (proprioception) and improves the "relaxation-contraction" coordination. This type of stretching is appropriate prior to beginning any activity and must be included as part of the provided warm-up. See warm-up section earlier in this chapter.

Slow, Static Stretching

Hold each static stretch for a minimum of 30 seconds and repeat each stretch a minimum of two times. Be progressive in your stretching. Exhale as you stretch farther into the range and then breathe normally as you hold the stretch at the point of tightness.

Key Areas

- Focus on muscles that tend to be relatively short and stiff: hamstrings, hip flexors, pectorals and quadriceps.
- Work with your physical therapist or personal trainer to determine which stretches are best for you.

Rules of Stretching

- Always warm up prior to stretching.
- Do dynamic stretching before each training session.
- Do static stretching as a separate session or during cooldown.

- Move slowly and smoothly into the stretch to avoid initiation of the stretch reflex (when the muscles tighten up to protect themselves if the stretch is too fast).
- Use proper body mechanics and strive for correct alignment.
- Regularly self-monitor optimal range of motion.
- Anticipate and communicate when stretching with a partner.
- Take one day off stretching per week.

Specific Stretching Tips

- Double knees to chest (spinal roll)—splay legs on either side of your abdomen to avoid uncomfortable compression
- Forearms—be especially careful if you have any carpal tunnel problems such as pain and numbness
- Thoracic spine—try extending your upper back over a rolled towel or an exercise ball
- Breathe—don't hold your breath or you may become dizzy
- Avoid toe pointing because calves may cramp

- Don't over-stretch—as the level of the hormone relaxin increases in your body you will automatically gain flexibility. Take note of your pre-pregnancy flexibility and do not exceed it.
- Lying on your left side while stretching decreases the pressure of the uterus on the vena cava (vein that returns blood from legs).

Always Fire the Core and Sustain During Stretching

Before each exercise focus on the following:
- Contract the pelvic floor (Kegel).
- Contract the TA (lower abdominal).
- Remember to breathe.
- Keep knees soft if standing.

> **NOTE**
>
> *These stretching exercises are not exhaustive and you may add others based on your experience or on the advice of your healthcare or fitness professional.*

Static Stretches—Upper Body

Exhale and hold each of these upper body static stretches for 10–15 seconds and repeat 2–3 times.

Side Stretch

- Stand with your core fired and sustain, shoulders square and feet about shoulder-width apart.
- Keeping knees soft, slowly reach up and lean to one side.

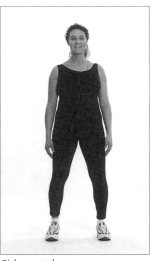
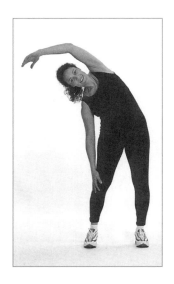

Side stretch.

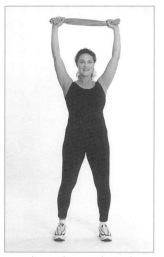 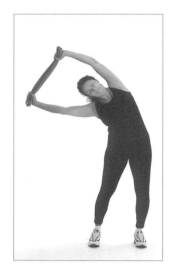

Standing side stretch (with towel).

Standing Side Stretch (with towel)

- Stand with your core fired and sustain, shoulders square and feet about shoulder-width apart.
- Grasp a towel with both hands over your head.
- Slowly bend from the waist, stretching your side.

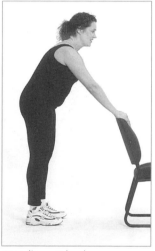 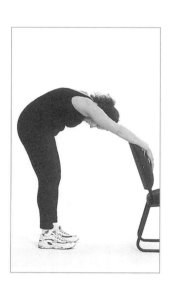

Standing cat back.

Standing Cat Back

- Stand with feet hip-width apart and hands on thighs, a chair or a countertop.
- Exhale while rounding back, pulling belly button toward spine. Fire the core and sustain.

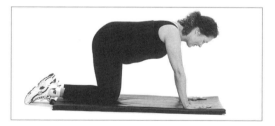

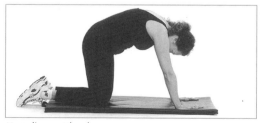

Kneeling cat back.

Kneeling Cat Back

- Kneel on the floor on all fours.
- Exhale while rounding your back, pulling belly button toward spine.

Triceps Stretch

- With arms overhead, hold the elbow of one arm with the other hand.
- Gently pull behind your head, stretching triceps.

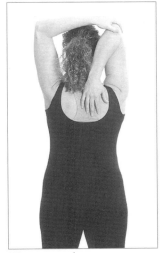

Triceps stretch.

Chest Stretch (Pectoral Stretch)

- Gently clasping hands behind back, press backward until you feel a stretch across your chest.

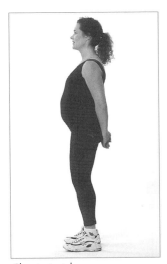

Chest stretch.

Chest Stretch Variation

- Place arm on wall with elbow bent at 90 degrees and below shoulder height.
- Push shoulder forward until you feel a stretch in your chest.

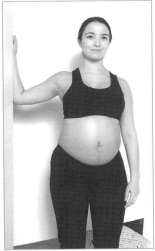

Chest stretch.

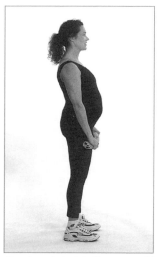
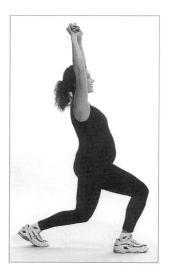

Overhead stretch (lunge position).

Overhead Stretch (lunge position with towel)

- Stand with your core fired and sustain, shoulders square and feet together.
- Holding a towel in both hands, take a small lunge step forward while raising your arms over your head.

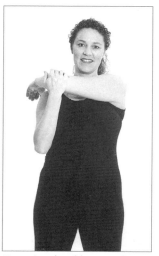

Posterior shoulder stretch.

Posterior Shoulder Stretch

- Gently pull your elbow across your chest toward the opposite side.
- If you feel pain in your shoulder, decrease the tension or stop the stretch.

Static Stretches—Lower Body

Exhale and hold each of these lower body static stretches for 20–40 seconds and repeat 2–3 times.

Quadriceps

- If you find it difficult to hold the foot to stretch, rest it on a chair or table (this prevents excessive compression under the kneecap). Standing, place the top of your foot on a stool or low table behind you.
- Hold onto a chair or table for balance.
- Keep a pelvic tilt, exhale and flex the front knee.
- To increase stretch place pillows under knee.

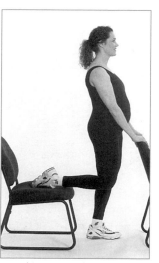

Quadricep stretch.

Hamstrings

- Place a rolled towel under your knee to avoid stressing the hamstring tendons on either side of the back of the knee.
- While standing next to a low table or chair, place straight leg on top, keeping hips square.
- Hold onto a chair or table for balance.
- Lean forward from waist and exhale, keeping chest up.

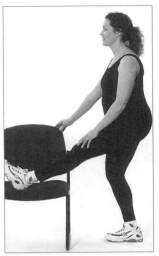

Hamstring stretch.

Seated Hamstring and Calf Stretch (towel assisted)

- *Go easy* or *avoid* to prevent cramping which can occur during pregnancy (point toe in and do both bent and straight knee).
- Sitting on the floor with your shoulders square, fire the core and sustain then bend from your hips as you gently pull the towel toward you.

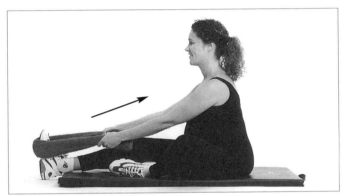

Seated hamstring and calf stretch.

Calves (Gastrocnemius-Soleus)

- Hold onto a chair or table for balance.
- Step forward with one foot and bend knee slightly, keeping rear leg straight.
- Keeping front heel down, bend forward until you feel a stretch behind the knee.
- Repeat with rear leg, pressing the heel down and feeling the stretch.

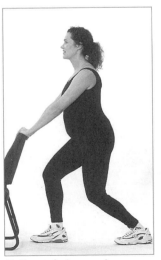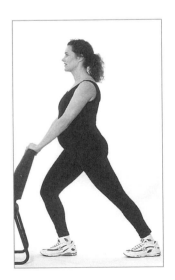

Calf stretch (go easy).

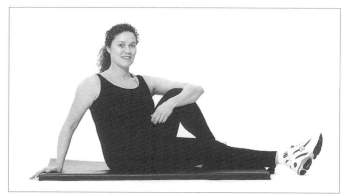

Hip abductor stretch.

Outer Thighs (Hip Abductors)

- Sit on the floor and cross one leg over the other so foot is flat on the floor at knee level.
- Rotate your torso so that opposite elbow touches outside of raised knee.
- Exhale and look over your shoulder as you stretch.

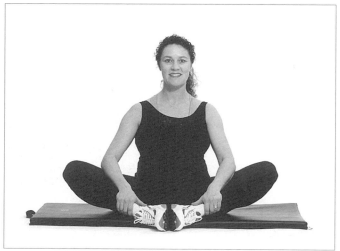

Hip adductor stretch.

Inner Thighs (Hip Adductors)

- *Go easy* as your pregnancy progresses due to the potential for irritating the attachments at the pubic bone.
- Do not perform this stretch in the third trimester—the pelvis "widens" to prepare for birth, making injury more likely.
- Sit upright on the floor with legs flexed up and heels close, letting knees fall toward the floor.
- Keep back straight. Try to balance even pressure on your sitting bones.

> **NOTE**
> *Avoid this stretch if you have any groin pain.*

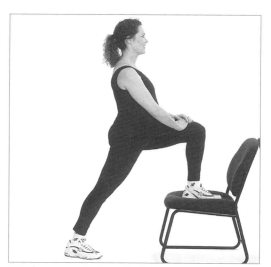

Hip flexor stretch (standing).

Hip Flexors (standing)

- Put one foot behind you and the other foot on a bench or chair.
- Allow knee to bend as you push your opposite hip forward, feeling the stretch at the front of the thigh.

Hip Flexors (kneeling)

- Kneel on the floor with one leg forward and push the back hip forward, feeling the stretch at the front of the thigh.

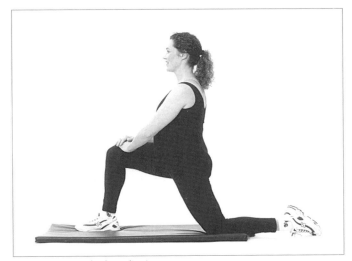

Hip flexor stretch (kneeling).

Knees to Chest (Paraspinal Roll)

- Lie flat on your back with knees bent (first trimester only—do left sidelying after).
- Bring both knees up toward chest and rock knees gently up, stretching low back and buttock muscles.

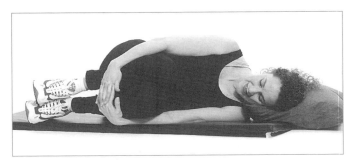

Knees to chest stretch.

Sidelying Knees to Chest

- Lie on your left side and exhale as you draw your knees to your chest.
- This is an excellent low back and buttock stretch for the second and third trimesters.
- Your rest position between stretches should be left sidelying.

What Happens to Your Body During Pregnancy?

Physiological Changes of Pregnancy

Pregnancy is a time of enormous physiological change. The adjustments that your body is required to make to nourish and carry a baby to term affect every major organ system. The significant changes are discussed below.

Cardiovascular System (Heart and Blood Vessels)

A woman's blood volume can increase by up to 50% during pregnancy; this occurs mainly between the sixth and twenty-fourth week. The heart's response to the greater blood volume is to increase both heart rate and stroke volume (the amount of blood the heart pumps out). As a result, the pregnant woman often has a higher heart rate at rest than her non-pregnant counterparts. This is

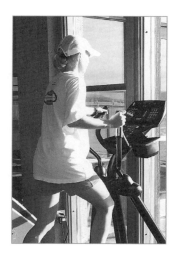

the reason that heart rate monitoring was abandoned in 1994 as a measure of exercise intensity in the pregnant woman. Instead, intensity should be measured by using the Borg Scale or talk test guidelines (see page 59).

The changes in blood volume also cause a change in blood pressure. The measured blood pressure in a pregnant woman is significantly lower than in her non-pregnant state, which is why you may often feel light-headed in early pregnancy.

Respiratory System (Lungs)

The increase in blood volume causes a greater demand for oxygen in the pregnant woman, and the body responds by increasing both the depth and frequency of respirations. You may often find yourself short of breath when you are pregnant; this is because your body is working much harder than before, even at rest.

Metabolism

To meet the demands of the growing baby your metabolism must change at its most basic level. The baby requires glucose (sugar) to grow and develop; as a result the body diverts glucose away from the tissues toward the placenta. The extra glucose requirement necessitates an increase in your caloric intake. It also causes the cells in your body to work harder than they did before pregnancy, releasing more energy which in turn is dissipated as heat. This extra heat may cause you to feel flushed and warm throughout most of your pregnancy. During exercise, the extra heat can actually be harmful to you and your baby if not safely released. It is important not to overheat during your exercise sessions, and to make sure you wear clothing that allows heat to dissipate quickly.

Cardiovascular activity is the mainstay of most fitness programs and the area in which most of the research in the field of exercise during pregnancy has been done. This research has shown that if you engaged in consistent cardiovascular activity prior to pregnancy, you can and should continue your exercise regime during pregnancy (Collings, Curet & Mullin, 1983; Hall & Kaufmann, 1987; Clapp, 1989; Clapp, 1996). Your first priority, however, is to shift your focus from training to simply maintaining your current fitness level. Your body is undergoing dramatic changes which will leave you feeling fatigued, so don't push yourself to the point of exhaustion. Your exercise program should be flexible and allow for modifications depending on your energy level each day—work harder if you're feeling well, take it easy if you're feeling tired or use that day to rest and recover.

If you have not exercised prior to pregnancy you can begin a low-intensity walking program or a prenatal exercise class that is taught by a qualified instructor. Gradually increase the duration of your workout but be sure not to overexert yourself.

Intensity level is very important during pregnancy. Because of the physical changes in your body it is better to use perceived exertion rather than heart rate as a measure of intensity. The Borg Scale of Perceived Exertion follows; you should exercise in the 3 to 5 range. Another method of perceived exertion is the talk test; you should be able to carry on a conversation while you exercise, and if you cannot you should decrease your intensity.

Diversify Your Cardio Training

Everyone should have a diverse cardio program. For example, your program may use a mix of running, stationary cycling, swimming, pool running, elliptical training or stairclimbing to achieve aerobic fitness. Besides offering a greater range of alternatives for the fitness enthusiast, diversity of training promotes development of fundamental skills and helps to normalize muscle balance that may be negatively affected by pregnancy. In addition, you may find some activities more suitable at different stages of pregnancy; for example, cycling may be fine in the first trimester but uncomfortable in

Borg Scale of Perceived Exertion		Talk Test Guidelines
0	Nothing at all	Can very easily carry on a conversation
1	Very easy	
2	Easy	
3	Moderate	Should be able to carry on a conversation
4	Somewhat hard	
5	Hard	
6		Can't talk continuously
7	Very hard	
8		Can't talk at all
9		
10	Very, very heavy (maximal)	

the third. By cross-training throughout, you will never feel like you have to give up an activity.

Sport and Exercise Cautions

If you exercised prior to pregnancy you should be able to continue most exercise programs throughout your pregnancy, with a few modifications. It is important to remember that the baby leaves the protection of the pelvis by the fifteenth week and is therefore more susceptible to trauma. As well, your center of gravity shifts throughout pregnancy, putting you at greater risk of falling. Sports that may result in falls or abdominal trauma, such as cycling, skiing or horseback riding, should be avoided after the fifteenth week. You may find certain exercises increasingly uncomfortable as pregnancy progresses, due to weight gain or the manner in which you are carrying the child; for example, many women find running difficult in their last trimester. If you are a runner, remember that you can move your workout to the pool or switch to walking to maintain fitness. Competitive sports that involve impact or contact (even accidental) to the abdominal area such as soccer, basketball, hockey or other team sports should be approached with caution. Remember, it is not your skill but the skill of others that may put you at risk. As well, the competitive environment surrounding many team sports may tempt you to push yourself too far. Sports that involve sudden changes in speed or direction should also be avoided.

Traditional aerobics classes are, in general, safe. Keep in mind that you may need to modify intensity or moves as your pregnancy progresses. Exercise caution in a fitness class as often a "group" mentality takes over and you work harder than you are able, which can be especially dangerous during pregnancy.

The following moves are difficult for a pregnant woman and should be avoided:
• back hyperextensions
• deep leg press, lunges or squats (go to 70 degrees only)
• step-ups greater than 70 degrees
• fast interval training
• plyometrics (hopping or bounding exercises)
• crossing elbows to knees (your expanding abdomen is often in the way)
• supine (lying on your back) exercising for more than 30 seconds in trimesters two and three
• lateral raises above 70 degrees
• military press or overhead press.

Walking

This workout can be done outside or on a treadmill. Make sure you have a good pair of athletic shoes that allow for the increase in width and length of foot size, and that have adequate heel support. *Important:* Always use the talk test and/or rate of perceived exertion during your exercise sessions.

TIPS FROM THE TEAM

• Wear sturdy supportive shoes.
• Dress for the weather. Remember not to overheat. Dress in layers.
• Make use of nature's stairclimber by tackling the local hills.
• Change your route, intensity or length of workout for variety and to ensure a good overall workout that's fun and varied.
• Remember to work in your comfortable talk test range.

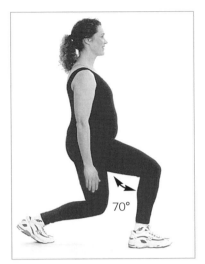

Lunges.

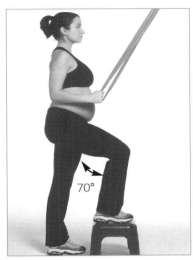

Step-ups.

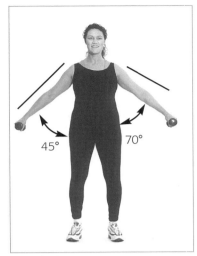

Lateral raises.

WALKING WORKOUT		
	First Trimester	**Second Trimester**	**Third Trimester**
Beginner	You were new to exercise prior to pregnancy. Start by walking at an easy pace for 30 minutes, 2–3 times per week, with a day of rest in between.	Begin to increase the intensity of your walk. Warm up by walking briskly for 5–10 minutes, then pick up the pace and power walk (walking at a fast pace, pumping your arms) for 25 minutes. Cool down by walking slowly for 5 minutes. Do this 2–3 times per week.	After 5 minutes of walking briskly, aim to power walk for 30 minutes, followed by a cooldown of 5 minutes of walking slowly. If you aren't up to the intensity, ride a recumbent bike or use a stair-climber. Stick to flat terrain. Try to walk at least twice a week.
Intermediate	You were power walking (walking at a fast pace, pumping your arms) consistently for at least 3 months prior to pregnancy for 45 minutes, 3–4 times per week. Continue this routine, making sure to take a day of rest in between.	If everything went well in your first trimester and you're feeling up to it, continue at the same pace or increase to 4 times per week. Decrease pace if you feel tired, to a 10-minute warm-up, 30 minutes of power walking and a 10-minute cooldown.	Continue the 2nd trimester routine if you are still comfortable. Stick to flat terrain. If you need to decrease mileage, cross-train or work out in a pool to maintain your fitness level.
Advanced	You were power walking (walking at a fast pace, pumping your arms) consistently for 6 months or more prior to pregnancy for 1 hour, 4–5 times per week. You can continue this routine, but do not overexert yourself.	If everything went well in your first trimester and you're feeling up to it, continue at the same pace or increase to 5 times per week. Decrease pace if you feel tired, to a 10-minute warm-up, 40 minutes of power walking and a 15-minute cooldown.	Continue the 2nd trimester routine if you are still comfortable. Stick to flat terrain. If you need to decrease mileage, cross-train or work out in a pool to maintain your fitness level.

WALK-RUN PROGRAM			
	Walk (minutes)	Jog (minutes)	Total Workout (minutes)
Week 1			
Day 1	4.5	0.5	20–30
Day 2	4.0	1.0	20–30
Day 3	3.5	1.5	20–30
Week 2			
Day 1	4.0	1.0	20–30
Day 2	3.5	1.5	20–30
Day 3	3.0	2.0	20–30
Week 3			
Day 1	3.5	1.5	20–30
Day 2	3.0	2.0	20–30
Day 3	2.5	2.5	20–30
Week 4			
Day 1	3.0	2.0	20–30
Day 2	2.5	2.5	20–30
Day 3	2.0	3.0	20–30
Week 5			
Day 1	2.0	3.0	20–30
Day 2	1.5	3.5	20–30
Day 3	1.0	4.0	20–30
Week 6			
Day 1	1.5	3.5	20–30
Day 2	1.0	4.0	20–30
Day 3	0.5	4.5	20–30

TIPS FROM THE TEAM

- Don't push yourself.
- Drink enough water—drink to thirst.
- Fuel up—eat to appetite.
- Don't overheat.

Walk-Run Program

Do a dynamic warm-up and lightly stretch all leg muscles (see chapter 5). Start with fast walking daily until you are able to walk continuously for 45 minutes, 3 days in a row, with no pain or stiffness. Then start Week 1 of the program, leaving a day in between to rest.

After week 6 you should be able to jog continuously for 20 to 30 minutes. Increase gradually.

Stationary Cycling

Always use the talk test and/or rate of perceived exertion during your exercise sessions. Before beginning these suggested workouts ensure that you have warmed up adequately; try the dynamic warm-ups listed in chapter 5. If your trimester guidelines and fitness level do not allow 30 minutes in one training session or you are feeling tired, you may shorten the cardio portion of your workout to a more suitable length.

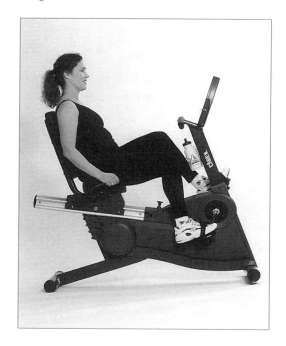

Stairclimber and Rowing

Always use the talk test and/or rate of perceived exertion during your exercise sessions. Before beginning these suggested workouts ensure that you have warmed up adequately; try the dynamic warm-ups listed in chapter 5. If your trimester guidelines and fitness level do not allow 30 minutes in one training session or you are feeling tired, you may shorten the cardio portion of your workout to a more suitable length.

You may also choose to do a full 15–30 minutes on any one piece of cardio equipment. Try not to use the same piece of equipment exclusively; variety will help keep you motivated.

	Time (minutes)	Program	RPE
A	30	Random	3
B	6	Warm-up	3
	24	Hill profile	3–5
C	5	Warm-up (manual)	3
	1	1–2 levels higher	3–4
	6	Same level as warm-up	3
	2	1–2 levels higher	3–4
	7	Same level as warm-up	3
	3	1–2 levels higher	3–4
	6–10	Same level as warm-up	3

SAMPLE WORKOUTS AEROBIC PROGRAMS

	Cardio Machine	Time (minutes)	RPE
A	Elliptical trainer	8–12	3
	Rower	8–12	3
	Stairclimber	8–12	3
B	Stairclimber	10–15	3
	Elliptical trainer	10–15	4
C	Rower	10–15	4
	Stairclimber	10–15	4

SAMPLE WORKOUTS MIXED CARDIO MACHINES

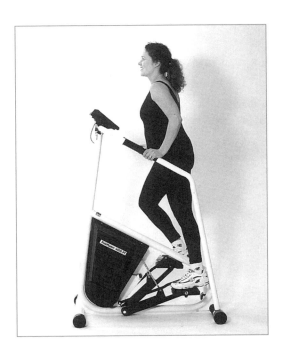

TIPS FROM THE TEAM

- Try a smooth track or treadmill for better shock absorption.
- Soft smooth terrain is ideal. Avoid rough, uneven terrain or slippery conditions.
- Avoid steep uphills as they may tempt you to push your intensity level too far.
- Avoid downhills due to the increased weight on the joints.

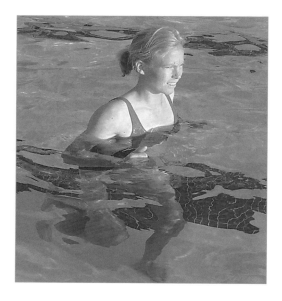

Water Workouts

Water workouts are a refreshing way to change and update your usual fitness routine, and it is easy to transfer land-based workouts into a non-weight-bearing environment. Water supplies three-dimensional resistance for strength-type movements while providing the buoyancy necessary to ease the stress on joints and muscles caused by most cardio routines. As well as adding resistance, water workouts also work the core stabilizers as your core muscles must work full time to maintain your balance and upright position. Another benefit can be a temporary reduction in leg swelling.

The IDEA Health and Fitness Association provides these suggestions for bringing workouts like running, cycling and aerobics into the pool.

- Understand how water impacts your body.
- What works on land doesn't always work in water.
- While gravity pulls the body downward on land, water's buoyancy pushes the body upward.

- Water's heaviness provides resistance to every movement, and this resistance increases exponentially with movement speed.

General Guidelines

Choose the right water depth, as this will affect how much weight you are bearing. Shallow water (generally, above the waist to chest-high) is suitable for water aerobics, gymnastics and yoga because the feet support the action. Shallow water is fine if you are quite fit or in the early stages of pregnancy, when you can tolerate more resistance from gravity on your joints. If the water level is above the chest you are essentially in a non-weight-bearing environment.

Modify your moves for the water. When doing resistance training perform moves at one-half to one-third the speed you would on land; your effort will be the same or even greater. Conversely, when jogging in deep water try to keep a pace similar to that on land. When jogging or walking in shallow water, slow the upper-body moves to match those of the lower body, which needs time to press through the water.

> **NOTE**
> *The chlorine in a pool, which helps keep the pool free of bacteria, will not harm you or your baby.*

Water Jogging

Water jogging is an excellent low-impact workout. With the weight and size gain during pregnancy your joints and muscles will appreciate the buoyancy of the water. An easy jog can act as a natural massage and helps soothe fatigue or tightness in the muscles, all the while working the muscles through the resistance of the water. In order to maintain fitness you will need to exercise with the same intensity, duration and frequency as you would on land.

Mastering the Basics

- For your first few sessions, wear a flotation device around your waist that will allow you to comfortably keep your head above water in the deep end of the pool—your feet should not be touching the bottom. Begin to jog by mimicking your running style on land: keep your body upright and avoid bending at the waist. Drive your knee forward to about a 45-degree angle; extend your leg to allow your heel to plant first, then flex your ankle so that you simulate pushing off the ground with your toes as you drive your leg back behind you, and the opposite leg begins the cycle once again. Make sure to pump your arms as if you were running on land.

Maintaining Good Form

- Avoid making a "bicycling" motion with your legs. Extend your quadriceps forward rather than upward, and concentrate on using your hamstrings to pull the water back behind you. Just as you cup the water with your hand when you do the front crawl, the idea is to "cup" the water with your hamstrings as your leg finishes the running motion.
- Hold your wrists straight and your fingers relaxed—don't cup your hands and do a "dog paddle" arm motion to stay afloat.
- Resist the tendency to lean forward and become more horizontal. As an easy check, when you look down you should be able to see your knees coming up in front of you.
- Don't sacrifice proper technique for speed. Move through the water slowly and steadily, and concentrate on your good form.

Water Jogging Tips

- Start slowly. Structure your program so that you gradually progress toward longer workouts. Before diving into hard workouts, you should be able to comfortably handle a steady 20- to 30-minute run.
- Make your workout as pleasant as possible. Find a pool with a large deep end or diving tank that is available at convenient times and not overly crowded. Music really helps pass the time as you work out.
- Find a partner. Arrange to meet and go for a run at the pool. Good conversation also helps pass the time.
- Keep time. Use a waterproof watch to time your runs and intervals, or find a pool with a large pace clock.
- Stop if you feel chilled or fatigued.

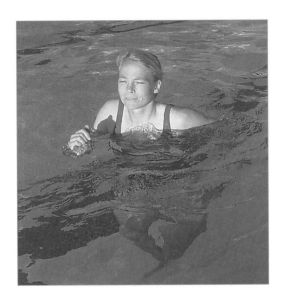

As you get more comfortable with deep water running, try doing portions of your workout without the flotation device. Continue to focus on form and if you feel that you are sinking, put the flotation device back on.

Water Workouts—Sample Routines

- Adjust based on your fitness level.
- Remember to start any new activity slowly and at a low intensity, and increase slowly.
- Warm up with some walking, and leg and arm swings.

Cardio Endurance

Run in deep water, at a consistent speed, for as long as you would run on land. The effort should be within your talk test range. Use cadence as an indicator of your effort; imagine your normal cadence on land and transfer this to the pool.

Tempo runs are a great way to increase your endurance. Start with 10 minutes of a normal pace followed by 10 minutes of an increased tempo. Keep the increased tempo at a pace that you can maintain, but your effort should be a step up from your regular jog pace. Finish with 10 minutes of a regular jog pace.

Try a session where you use the flotation belt for only a portion of the run, or not at all.

Sample Water Running Workouts

Your routine should include longer intervals of 1–3 minutes with rest periods of easy treading water, or rest on the side of the pool for 1–2 minutes between. Keep within your talk test range or an RPE of 3–5.

A. Do 5 × 3 minutes with 1–2 minutes recovery between each interval.

B. Do jogs of 5 minutes, 4 minutes, 3 minutes, 2 minutes and 1 minute with 1–2 minutes recovery.

C. Do 6 × 2 minutes with 1–2 minutes recovery.

D. Do 10 × 1 minute with 1 minute recovery.

Speed Play

- Warm up with 10 minutes of easy deep water jogging.
- Do 5 × 20 seconds fast (RPE = 5), with slow treading water for 1 minute between each set (RPE = 2–3).
- Run at an RPE of 4–5 for 30/45/60/75/90/75/60/45/30 seconds with a rest interval of about 50% of your run time.
- Do fast runs—2 sets of 3 × 60 seconds (RPE = 4–5)—with a rest interval of 30 seconds.
- Cool down with 10 minutes of easy water jogging.

Faster Runs (waist- to shoulder-deep water)

- Start with an easy jog for 5 minutes (RPE = 3–4).
- Do alternating leg walking lunges 2 × 10.
- Do high knees run (in shallow end) 6 × 1–2 minutes—rest interval is 30 seconds (RPE = 5).
- Do a ladder run: 2 sets of 30/45/60/45/30 seconds—rest interval is the same as work time (RPE = 5).
- Run heeling (heels to butt) 4 × 10–30 seconds (RPE = 4).
- Cool down by walking in the shallow end for 4 minutes (RPE = 2).

Water Walking (for those unable to swim)

- Warm up by walking back and forth and side to side 2–4 steps.
- Continue walking, swinging arms back and forth and in a figure-8 pattern to warm up the upper body.
- Add in shoulder shrugs with neck motion. Hang onto the side and do leg swings. Do walking crossovers, keeping high knees and stiff shoulders.
- Bob up and down for 10–20 seconds and repeat 2 × 4 times.
- Try walking forward 8 steps and backward 4. To increase resistance keep palms flat against direction of pull.
- Try some on-the-spot jogging in waist- to chest-deep water. Add in high knees and high heel kicks.
- Try some water stepping on a low step.

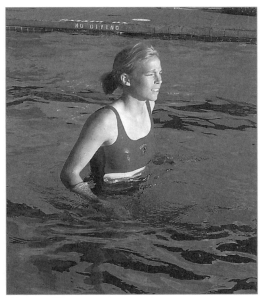
Water walking.

Water Strengthening

- Most pools run water aerobics and water strengthening classes using flotation belts, pool noodles, foam dumbbells and other resistance aids.
- Torso Twists—Standing with bent knees in the pool, do a pelvic tighten and side bend to the right and left side, holding each stretch for 4–6 seconds. Do some torso twists to the right and left, ensuring head follows shoulder. Do not over-stretch.
- Leg Workout—Try doing some split squats, 1/3 squats, and hip work flexion, abduction, adduction and extension. Do several sets of 10–20 repetitions.
- Shoulder and Torso Strength (shoulder-deep water)—Using tools such as fins, paddles and webbed gloves increases the

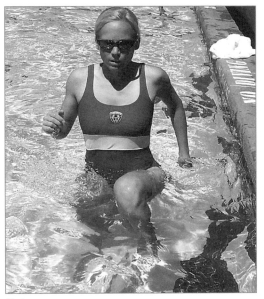
Faster runs.

surface area and resistance. Practice forehand- and backhand-like swing motions with both your dominant and non-dominant hands. Use a correct low-high swing and concentrate on technique. Try doing 2–3 sets of 15–20 strokes.
- Pool Press—Stand in shoulder-deep water with knees bent, or straddle a pool noodle.

Extend your arms in front on the water surface and sweep arms forward and backward, using the palms for resistance. Do 10–20 repetitions.

- Leg Diamonds—Wrap a pool noodle around your back and under your arms. Float in the water with knees apart and the soles of your feet touching, legs in a diamond shape. Lift legs up and down as you tighten tummy using the water's resistance to strengthen abdominals and legs. Do 10–20 repetitions.

Swimming

Swimming is a great exercise for pregnancy. It's a whole body workout without the pounding, straining or twisting often found in land-based activities.

Safety Tips

- Never swim alone.
- Be careful around the pool edge, as it is slippery.
- Use the steps or ladder to get in and out.
- Do not dive or jump in while you are pregnant.
- Avoid crowded pools where you may be elbowed or kicked.
- Stop swimming if you feel too hot, too cold or too tired.
- Be sure to drink plenty of water during your pool workout.

Stroke Selection

Choose the stroke you are most comfortable with and proficient at. Ensure you are breathing properly so you don't run out of breath and fatigue more quickly.

- *Crawl*—Recommended throughout pregnancy. It works both the right and left side equally. Ensure proper breathing.
- *Breaststroke*—Good throughout pregnancy because you can decrease the intensity as your pregnancy progresses, and you are able to see where you are going and keep your head out of the water to breathe more regularly. Exercise caution if you have back problems due to increased lordosis of the low back, knee problems or groin (symphysis pubis) pain.
- *Backstroke*—A good stroke, especially if you find breathing difficult with your forearms in the water. Be careful because you cannot see where you are going. Use different arm strokes (alternate sculling and crawl) to work different muscles.
- *Sidestroke*—Good throughout pregnancy, as it allows easy breathing and you can see where you are going. Ensure equal time is spent on each side.

These are just a few examples of water workouts. Regardless of fitness level, the water affords athletes a different playing field in which to train or recover. Don't worry if you feel a little sluggish when you get back on land for a regular workout; this feeling will disappear quickly. For more water workout ideas consult a reputable physical therapist or aquatics instructor who has experience working with pregnant women.

Nordic Walking

Nordic walking is a great cross-training fitness exercise that is a suitable alternative for women either before, during or after pregnancy. It can be a very good workout for pregnant women who want to stay in shape and benefit from an upper body workout as well. Nordic walking uses two poles (designed for walking) to work the upper body while walking or hiking. Like cross-country skiing, the poles are used by the arms to match each step you take, giving a better overall workout without feeling like you are working any harder. While you can get a similar effect simply by walking faster, many pregnant women do not want to or cannot walk faster. On any surface, proper use of the poles and arm motion encourages good posture and provides more stability for pregnant women who often have balance or low back and hip concerns.

Getting Started

Correct pole length for exercising is calculated by using the simple formula of your height × .68. Pole lengths are graded in 5 cm intervals, so the calculated ideal length should be rounded off to the nearest 5 cm (best to go to the shortest length). The rule of thumb is that a Nordic walker's elbow should be at approximately a 90-degree angle when holding the grip with the tip of the pole on the ground. If you are new to Nordic walking you may find that having a slightly shorter pole length is easier.

Suggested Benefits of Nordic Walking

- Energy consumption increases by an average of 20% compared with ordinary walking without poles.
- It is estimated that 80–90% of all muscles of the body are used when Nordic walking.
- Helps improve posture and decrease posture problems associated with pregnancy.

- Helps relieve muscle tension in the neck and shoulder region by working the muscles rhythmically.
- Helps improve lateral mobility of the neck and spine.
- The upper body muscles most actively involved are the forearm extensor and flexor muscles, the posterior shoulder muscles, the large pectorals and the upper back muscles.
- Use of poles as a balance and propulsion aid helps minimize stress on the ankle, knee and hip joints.
- Caloric expenditure is approximately 400 calories per hour (compared with 280 calories per hour for normal walking).
- Use of poles helps increase the safety factor on slippery surfaces and can aid balance as the pregnancy progresses.
- Ensure good quality walking, running or hiking shoes.
- Ensure proper clothing, and dress in layers with fabrics that breathe.

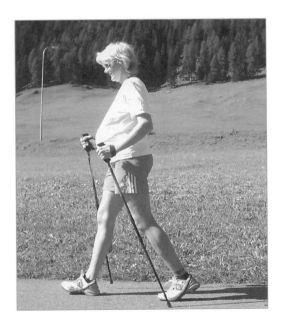

Technique Tips

The technique is a simple enhancement of normal arm swing when walking. The poles remain behind and pointing diagonally backward at all times.

- Shoulders should remain relaxed and down.

> **NOTE**
>
> *Keeping the arms relaxed and keeping the poles behind the body are key elements in the proper technique.*

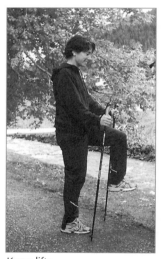

Knee lifts.

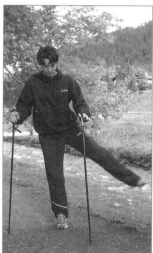

Leg swings.

- Keep poles held close to the body.
- The hands are opened slightly to allow the poles to swing forward (the poles are not gripped but swing from the wrist straps).
- As the leading foot strikes the ground the opposite arm swings forward to waist height.
- The opposite pole strikes the ground, level with the heel of the opposite foot.
- The poles remain pointing diagonally backward, never in front of the body.
- Push the pole as far back as possible, straightening the arm at the end of the swing. The hand lets go of the grip.
- Remember the length of the steps is greater than traditional steps allowing the arms enough time to finish the movement.
- The foot rolls through the step to push off with the toe. This lengthens the stride behind the body, getting the most out of each stride.
- The arm motion stays loose and relaxed.

Sample Warm-up Exercises

Knee Lifts

- Stand with poles on each side.
- Keep back straight and core fired at all times.
- Pull knee up to 90 degrees.
- Repeat 1–2 × 10 repetitions per leg.

Leg Swings

- Stand with poles on each side.
- Keep back straight and core fired at all times.
- Keep the supporting leg slightly bent.
- Swing one leg out to the side to 30–45 degrees.
- Repeat 1–2 × 10 repetitions per leg.

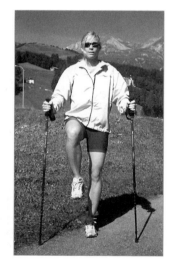

Torso Twists (back and shoulder)

- Stand with a wide stance.
- Place poles in hand over head onto shoulders.
- Keep the knees slightly bent and core fired.
- Gently twist torso to rotate right and left.
- Repeat 1–2 × 6 repetitions per direction.

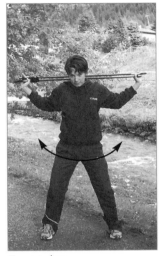

Torso twists.

Adductor Stretch

- Stand with a wide stance, poles out in front and in the middle of your body.
- Fire the core and sustain.
- Lunge laterally to one side keeping one leg straight.
- Keep back straight but bent slightly forward.
- Repeat 1–2 × 10 repetitions per leg.
- *Caution:* Do not stretch aggressively after 24 weeks or if you have groin pain at any time in pregnancy.

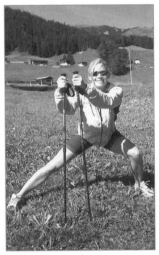
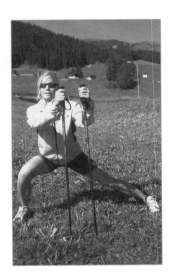

Adductor stretch.

Sample Strength Exercises

Pole Squats

- Stand with poles out in front and on each side.
- Fire the core and sustain.
- Bend knees down to 45–90 degrees (not lower).
- Keep back straight but bent slightly forward.
- Repeat 1–2 × 10 repetitions per leg.

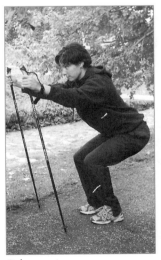
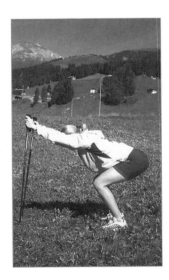

Pole squats.

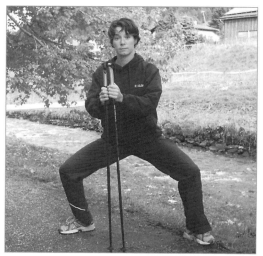

Sumo pole squats.

Sumo Pole Squats

- Stand with a wide stance, poles out in front and in the middle of your body.
- Fire the core and sustain.
- Bend knees down to 45–90 degrees (not lower).
- Keep back straight but bent slightly forward.
- Repeat 1–2 × 10 repetitions per leg.

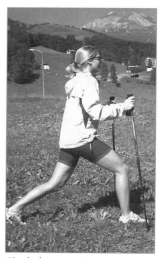
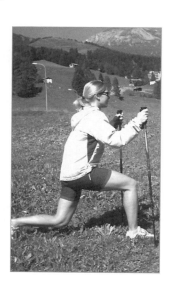

Single leg squats.

Single Leg Squats

- Stand with poles out in front and on each side of you.
- Keep back straight, and fire the core and sustain.
- Step forward with one leg until in a split squat position.
- Bend down slowly on one leg, not going lower than 90 degrees.
- Repeat 1–2 × 10 repetitions per leg.

Many Nordic walking routines advocate doing different types of hops and jumps, either side to side or front and back. It is best to avoid these while pregnant as they may place too much stress on your joints. However, once your strength and stability have increased postpartum you can try slowly adding some for variety. As always, consult your healthcare professional before beginning any new exercise program.

> **NOTE**
>
> With the poles to aid balance and using your imagination you can do a number of other stretches for the legs, arms and torso. See chapter 5 for more ideas.

Sample Program—Beginners

Nordic walking program for beginners and pregnant women

If you are planning on incorporating Nordic walking into your fitness routine and have not recently done any walking or running for fitness, start slowly. Those with a poor fitness level can begin by simply walking 8 × 10 minutes in 3 weeks. If you have an average to good fitness level you can start with Nordic walking right away. Add it in as you feel comfortable with other forms of exercise but ensure you accumulate an average of 40 to 60 minutes of activity, 4 to 6 times per week.

More general information on Nordic walking can be found at www.nordicwalking.com.

Week 1	Start walking slowly and try to walk with your whole foot; on every step you should roll it from your heel to the toes. The arms are loose at your sides. Use poles easily, and don't force it.	10 min.
	Walk 15 minutes and try to get a good rhythm with poles and legs. Always use right leg and left arm with pole at the same time.	15 min.
Week 2	Walk 2 × 10 minutes with a 2 minute break.	22 min.
	Walk 2 × 12 minutes with a 2 minute break.	26 min.
Week 3	Walk 20 minutes and watch your RPE and breathing.	20 min.
	Walk 25 minutes.	25 min.
Week 4	Walk 2 × 12 minutes with a 2 minute break.	24 min.
	Walk 2 × 10 minutes with a 2 minute break. Try to walk the first 10 minutes faster.	22 min.
	Walk 25 minutes.	25 min.
Week 5	Walk 2 × 15 minutes with a 2 minute break.	32 min.
	Walk 2 × 15 minutes with a 2 minute break. Try to walk the first 15 minutes faster.	32 min.
	Walk 30 minutes.	30 min.
Week 6	Walk 2 × 15 minutes with a 5 minute break. Try to walk faster than normally both times.	35 min.
	Walk 35 minutes.	35 min.
	Walk 2 × 20 minutes with a 5 minute break.	45 min.

7

Strength or Resistance Training

Musculoskeletal System

During the sixth week of pregnancy the placenta begins to secrete a hormone called relaxin. The purpose of this hormone is to increase the elasticity of the ligaments in the pelvis, making it easier for the baby to move down through the pelvis at the time of delivery. Relaxin is not specific to the pelvis, however, and its effects can be demonstrated in all major joints of the body.

In response to relaxin, your joints can be more flexible than in your non-pregnant state. It is important not to overstretch during your workout, or you may damage your joints. The effects of relaxin are discussed in chapter 3, The Core.

Strength training is an essential component of any fitness program, and it is especially important for pregnant women. During pregnancy your body and center of gravity are changing continually, causing an increased lumbar curvature and leading to poor posture. Strength training allows you to strengthen the weak muscles and stretch the tight ones, which will help bring you back to a normal posture and decrease low back pain. Other benefits include increased muscle strength and tone, increased energy, improved flexibility and endurance, and reduced shoulder and neck strain. On a practical note, increased upper body strength will come in handy after your baby arrives as you find yourself toting the baby, diaper bag and groceries all at the same time.

If you were on a strength and conditioning program prior to pregnancy you can continue it throughout your pregnancy, with a few modifications. Due to the size of the developing baby, it is recommended that you avoid exercising in the supine position (on your back) after the third month of pregnancy (ACOG, 2002). Incline benches are great substitutes for flat bench exercises when you are using free weights. Due to increased joint laxity you should pay special attention to ensuring that you do not go past a normal range of motion in your exercises with free weights. Weight machines are normally designed to prevent this and can be a wonderful alternative during pregnancy.

If you have not been following a strength and conditioning program prior to pregnancy, you should seek an exercise prescription from an exercise physiologist, physical therapist or qualified prenatal professional.

To ensure postural stability, extra attention should be given to maintaining lower and upper back strength. Your strength and conditioning program should include all major muscle groups of the body.

A word on abdominal muscles: Although your abdomen is expanding it is still important to maintain good muscle tone. Abdominal exercises should not be done in the supine position after the first trimester of pregnancy. You can use an incline rather than a flat board, if you feel you have to perform traditional sit-ups. However, after reading about the core, we hope you have realized that by following the exercises and engaging your core in the process, you will not need traditional sit-ups now or in the future.

Smart Strength Training Guidelines

- Ensure good instruction and continued supervision.
- Warm up first (run, walk, cycle, etc.—see chapter 5, Warm-up).
- Before each exercise check the following:
  - When doing squats don't allow your knees to go past your toes (this increases pressure to undersurface of patella). Avoid deep squats (past 70 degrees).
  - Focus on proper technique (ask a knowledgeable health professional if you are unsure).
- Avoid overhead lifts (for example, military press) as they increase "hyperlordosis" or sway back.

- Avoid lateral arm raises (abduction) past 70 degrees.
- Perform your exercises in a slow and controlled manner.
- Start with light weights and increase gradually.
- Avoid heavy lifting throughout pregnancy (that is, don't lift excessively heavy weights, both inside and outside the gym). Now is not the time for attempting maximal lifts.

Always Fire the Core and Sustain

Before each exercise focus on the following:
- Contract the pelvic floor (Kegel).
- Contract the TA (lower abdominal).
- Remember to breathe.
- Keep knees soft if standing.

Selecting the Resistance

There are two ways to approach strength training: in the traditional form, with machines and free weights, or with resistance tubing. If you are using machines or free weights, you determine the resistance by trial and error (or get suggestions from a

---

TIPS FROM THE TEAM

- Always maintain good posture.
- Don't hyperextend (arch) your back while doing exercises.
- Fire the Core and Sustain (keep lower abdominal muscles switched on).
- Keep within your range of motion—now is not the time to increase flexibility.
- Breathe properly—exhale as you do the work.

CAUTION: *Do not hold your breath* while doing strength exercises. If any exercise position makes you feel dizzy or lightheaded it should be eliminated and an alternate exercise for that muscle group should be used.

physical therapist, exercise physiologist or qualified health professional). You should choose a weight that allows you to do 10 to 20 repetitions comfortably. If you can do only 6 reps, then decrease the resistance. It is an individualized system for training at your own rate and strength level. (Your strength level can vary from 10–20% over the course of a day, so adjust the resistance according to how you feel after the first set.)

With resistance tubing, you can perform the exercises slowly, and with proper form for a set amount of time or repetitions. Start with 30 seconds or 10 to 15 slow repetitions and work up to 1 minute; when that becomes too easy, choose tubing with more resistance.

> **NOTE**
>
> *These exercises are not exhaustive and you may add others based on your experience or on the advice of your healthcare or fitness professional.*

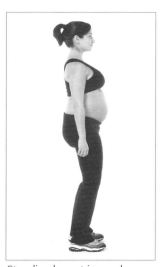 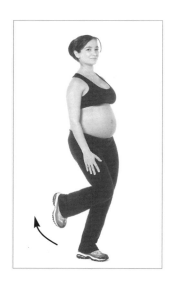

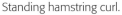
Standing hamstring curl.

Strength Training Guidelines

To make the exercises more difficult:

- Challenge your balance by performing the exercises on an exercise ball, ½ foam roll or Sissel disk; without any balance aid; or using free weights instead of a machine.
- Increase tension in the muscle by performing each move at a slow tempo, or by increasing the weight or strength of the resistance band.

Workout At Home

Even if you don't belong to a gym or have a Fit to Deliver class in your area, you can give your baby the benefits of exercise during pregnancy. By investing in a few simple pieces of equipment—some stretch cords, hand weights and an exercise ball—you can have your own home gym.

Before you start this sample exercise program be sure to warm up, and cool down after your workout (see chapter 5).

Always Fire the Core and Sustain

Before each exercise focus on the following:

- Contract the pelvic floor (Kegel).
- Contract the TA (lower abdominal).
- Remember to breathe.
- Keep knees soft if standing.

For each of the following exercises, perform 10–15 repetitions per side unless otherwise specified.

Standing Hamstring Curl

- Stand tall, and fire the core and sustain.
- Lift up one foot behind you and hold.
- Lower slowly.
- Strengthens hamstrings and buttocks.

Sidelying Abduction

- Lie on your left side, making sure your hips are stacked on top of each other.
- The left leg can be bent or straight, whichever is most comfortable.
- Rest your head on your left shoulder, or bend your left arm and cup your head in your hand.
- Fire the core and sustain.
- Raise your right leg 8–10 inches without rolling backward.
- Repeat on the opposite (right) side.
- Strengthens buttocks and hips.

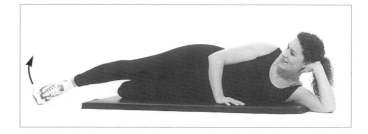

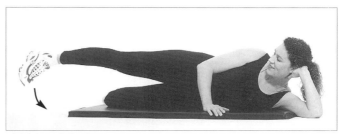

Sidelying abduction.

Sidelying Adduction

- Lie on your left side with your right hip and knee bent to 90 degrees and supported by a cushion or small step.
- Fire the core and sustain.
- Keeping your left leg straight, raise it up and hold.
- Repeat on opposite (right) side.
- Strengthens inner thighs.

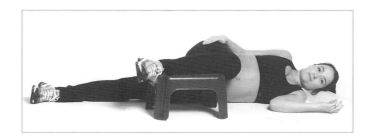

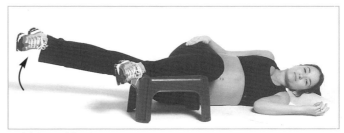

Sidelying adduction.

Sidelying Knee-ups

- Lie on your left side with your upper body propped under a pillow and your legs straight.
- Fire the core and sustain, and pull your knees toward your chest.
- Strengthens lower abdominals.

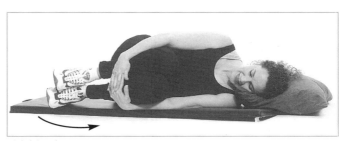

Sidelying knee-ups.

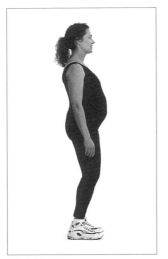
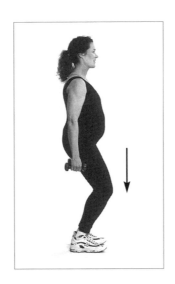

Mini (1/3) squats.

Mini (1/3) Squats

- Stand with your feet shoulder-width apart. Fire the core and sustain.
- Squat, and press your butt back like you are sitting in a chair.
- Lower yourself until you are about one-third of the way down to the chair.
- Start with no weight and add hand weights as needed.
- Strengthens quadriceps and buttocks.

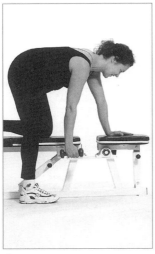
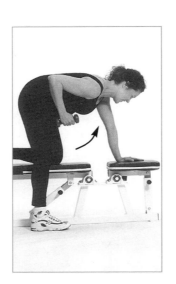

One arm row.

One-Arm Row

- Rest one arm and knee on a chair or bench.
- Keeping your back flat and your core fired, pull a weight or stretch cord (secured to the chair) back toward your hip.
- Strengthens lats and rhomboids.

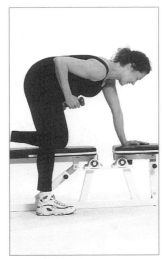
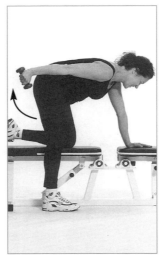

Tricep kickbacks.

Tricep Kickbacks

- Rest one arm and knee on a chair or bench.
- Keeping your back flat and your core fired, extend your arm backward.
- Be sure to keep your upper arm (bicep) pressed tight to your side and pivot from the elbow.
- Strengthens mid-back and triceps.

Bicep Curl and Lateral Raise (not shown)

- Sit in a chair with your arms at your sides.
- Curl your arms up to 90 degrees and then raise your arms laterally (out to the side).
- Ensure good shoulder posture.
- Strengthens biceps and shoulders.

Seated Knee Lift

- Sit on the edge of a chair with a pillow behind your back and feet on the floor, or sit on the floor leaning against a chair or wall.
- Lean back slightly, fire the core and sustain, and bend one knee up to your chest.
- Alternate legs, maintaining proper posture.
- Strengthens abdominals.

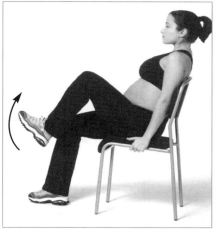

Seated knee lift.

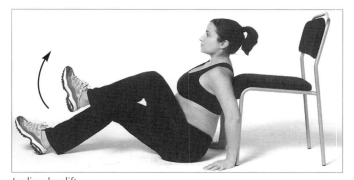

Incline leg lift.

Incline Fly

- Lie on your back, propped up against a couch, some pillows or an incline bench.
- Hold a dumbbell in each hand, arms out to the side.
- Keeping elbows slightly bent and palms facing in, bring your arms together above your chest until your hands touch.
- Strengthens chest, shoulders and triceps.

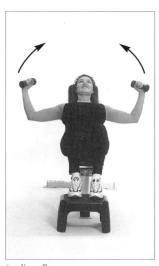 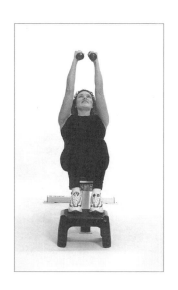

Incline fly.

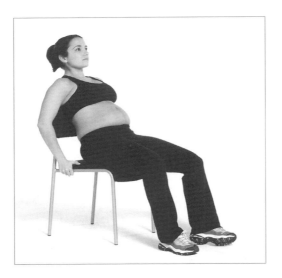

3-in-1 Incline Transverse Abdominal

- Lie on your back, propped up with pillows or blankets or lean back in a chair.
- Fire the core and sustain.
- Tighten and slide leg out and in, then tighten and let leg fall out to the side and back.
- Do this exercise in a slow and controlled manner.
- Strengthens lower abdominals.

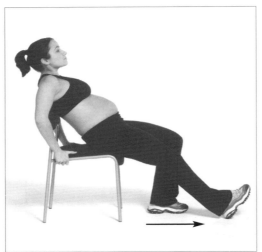

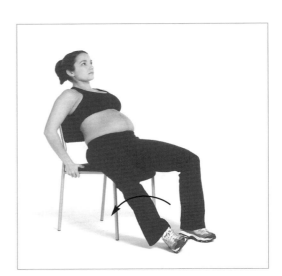

3-in-1 incline transverse abdominal.

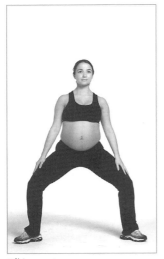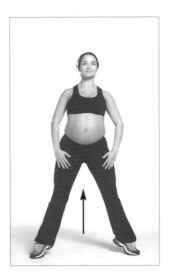

Plié squat.

Plié Squat

- Stand with your feet slightly apart and your toes pointed out.
- Fire the core and sustain.
- Do a plié mini squat, keeping your knees over your toes, then straighten your legs and rise up on your toes. (Avoid this exercise if you are prone to calf cramps.)
- Strengthens legs and hips.

Workout With Weights
Upper Body Strength Training
(Free Weights and Machines)

Familiarize yourself with the following exercises prior to beginning the program. These exercises are not exhaustive and you may add others based on your experience or on the advice of your healthcare or fitness professional.

Always Fire the Core and Sustain

Before each exercise focus on the following:

- Contract the pelvic floor (Kegel).
- Contract the TA (lower abdominal).
- Remember to breathe.
- Keep knees soft (slightly bent) if standing.

Flat Flys or Incline Flys

- Lie on your back (first trimester only) on a flat bench holding two dumbbells at arm's length above your shoulders. (For trimesters two and three, sit on an incline bench.)
- With your palms facing in, let your elbows bend slightly as you lower the weights out to the side until they are in line with your ears.
- Fire the core and sustain.
- Inhale as you return the weights to the starting position.
- Strengthens anterior chest and shoulders.

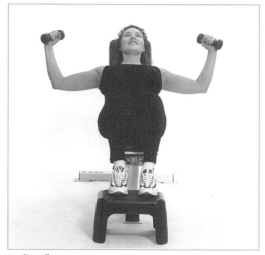
Incline flys.

Incline Bench Press (with stool)

- Sit on an incline bench, and fire the core and sustain.
- Place both feet on a stool so that your back is pressed against the bench.
- Hold a dumbbell in each hand with your elbows at your sides.
- Exhale as you extend your arms to the ceiling.
- Strengthens anterior chest and shoulders.

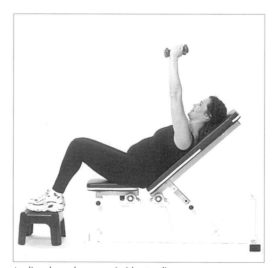
Incline bench press (with stool).

Lat Pulldowns (not shown)

- Sit down and hold the bar in a narrow (supinated) grip, palms facing you. (You can vary this exercise by using a pronated wide grip or a mid supinated grip.)
- Fire the core and sustain.
- Keeping your back straight, exhale as you pull the bar down to chest level.
- Inhale as you return your arms to the starting position.
- Strengthens mid back, posterior shoulder and biceps.

Seated Row (not shown)

- Sit on the seated row machine, fire the core and sustain, and keep shoulders down.
- Grasp the bar with both hands, palms facing down.
- Exhale as you bring your hands toward your chest.
- Strengthens mid back and posterior shoulder.

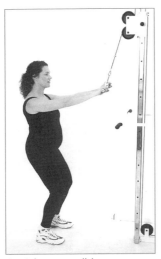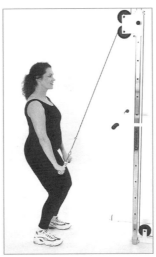

Straight arm pulldowns.

Straight Arm Pulldowns

- Stand facing the machine with your feet hip-width apart and shoulders square, then fire the core and sustain.
- Grasp the bar with both hands, shoulder-width apart, palms facing down.
- Keeping your arms straight but not locked, exhale as you bring your hands down to your thighs.
- Strengthens mid back and posterior shoulder.

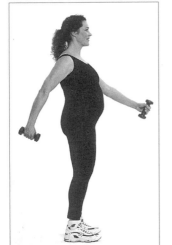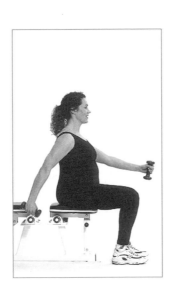

Front and back shoulder raises.

Front and Back Shoulder Raises (standing or seated)

- This can be done in the standing position with soft knees in the first trimester, and seated in the second and third trimesters.
- Keeping shoulders square, fire the core and sustain. Slowly raise one arm straight out in front of you to just below shoulder height.
- Alternate arms, keeping the movement under control the whole time.
- Strengthens anterior and posterior shoulder.

Lateral Raises (standing or seated)

- Hold a weight in each hand and exhale as you raise your arms to the side, never exceeding 70 degrees.
- Slowly lower weights to the starting position.
- Strengthens lateral shoulder.

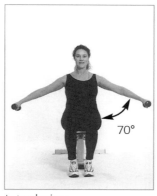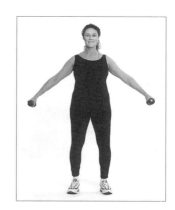

Lateral raises.

Bent Over Lateral Raises

- Sit on the side of a bench and bend forward from your hips as you fire the core and sustain.
- Hold a dumbbell in each hand, arms at your sides.
- Exhale as you raise your arms to the side, keeping your elbows slightly bent.
- As your pregnancy progresses move your feet farther apart so that your tummy can fit between your knees.
- Strengthens mid back and posterior shoulder.

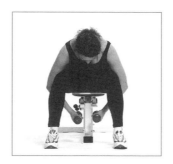

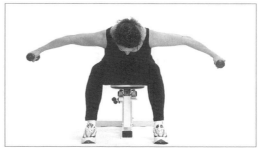

Bent over lateral raises.

Bicep Low Cable Curls One Arm (not shown)

- Face the machine with soft knees, fire the core and sustain, and keep hips square.
- Keep one hand at your side while the other holds the handle at 90 degrees.
- Exhale as you bring your wrist to your chest.

TIPS FROM THE TEAM

Variety is one key to success in following a training program. If you become bored, try changing the exercises each month.

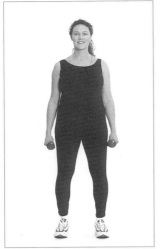
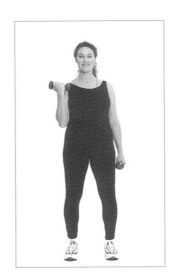

Bicep Curls (standing)

- Stand with your feet comfortably apart and knees slightly bent. Fire the core and sustain.
- With your palms facing forward, exhale as you curl your hands toward your shoulders.
- Inhale as you lower your hands to the starting position.
- Can be done alternating or both arms together.
- Strengthens biceps.

Bicep curls (standing).

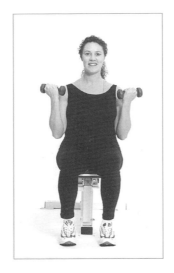

Bicep Curls (seated)

- Hold a dumbbell or a stretch cord in each hand, arms at your sides. Fire the core and sustain.
- With your palms facing forward, exhale as you curl your hands toward your shoulders.
- Inhale as you lower your hands to the starting position.
- Can be done alternating or both arms together.
- Strengthens biceps.

Bicep curls (seated).

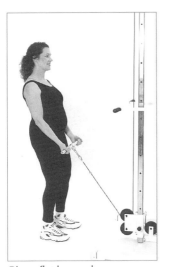
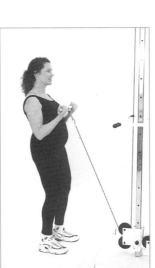

Bicep Flat Bar Curls

- Stand facing the machine with soft knees and hips square, then fire the core and sustain.
- Keeping your elbows at your sides, exhale as you bring your wrists to your chest.

Bicep flat bar curls.

Tricep Pressdowns (not shown)

- Stand in front of the lat pulldown bar with your feet shoulder-width apart. Hands are shoulder-width apart, palms down on the bar.
- Fire the core and sustain.
- With elbows at your sides, exhale as you press the bar down until your elbows are extended.
- Inhale as you slowly raise your hands toward your shoulders.
- Strengthens triceps and mid back.

> **TIPS FROM THE TEAM**
>
> - Make each repetition count.
> - Concentrate on performing each exercise correctly. Go slow and controlled.

Tricep Rope Pressdowns

- Stand in front of the machine with your knees soft, and fire the core and sustain.
- Start with your elbows at your hips, and bent at 90 degrees. Exhale as you press your hands down.
- Strengthens triceps and mid back.

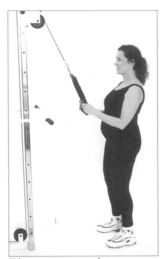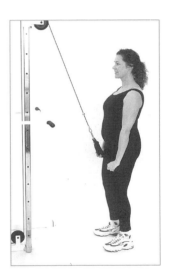

Tricep rope pressdowns.

Lower Body Strength Training (Free Weights and Machines)

Dumbbell Squats

- Standing with your feet hip-width apart, fire the core and sustain, arms hanging at your sides and holding dumbbells.
- Keep your back straight and head up, and look straight ahead.
- Inhale as you squat until your thighs are parallel to the floor.
- While squeezing your glutes and pushing with your quadriceps, exhale as you return to the starting position.
- Strengthens buttocks, thighs and core.

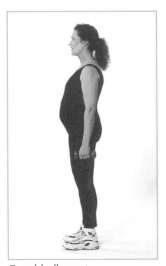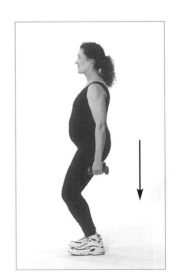

Dumbbell squats.

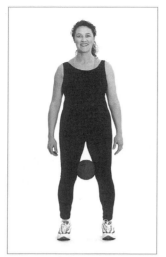
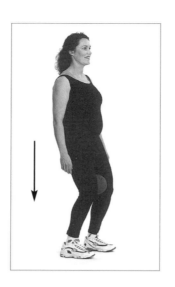

Squats with knee squeeze.

Squats with Knee Squeeze

- Stand tall, fire the core and sustain, and keep hips square.
- Hold a ball between your knees and lower yourself into a squat.
- You can do this exercise with your hands at your sides, or holding weights.
- Strengthens thighs and core, but targets inner thighs.

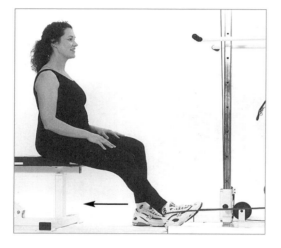

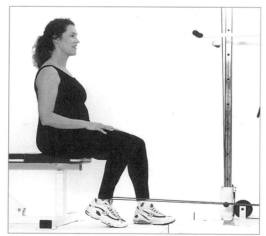

Seated hamstring curl.

Seated Hamstring Curl (cable or stretch cord)

- Sit on the machine with your feet out in front of you, ensuring that the heel cushion is at your ankles.
- Fire the core and sustain.
- Exhale as you draw your heels to your glutes, then inhale as you slowly return your legs to the starting position. Your back should remain neutral for the whole exercise.
- Strengthens posterior thighs and core.

TIPS FROM THE TEAM

- Don't sacrifice good form for more resistance or you may be setting yourself up for potential injury.
- Use a slow tempo or controlled movement through both the shortening and lengthening phases. If you use a machine don't bounce the weight stack.

Sidelying Leg Lifts

- Lie on your side, one hand supporting your head and opposite hand on the floor in front of your tummy.
- Fire the core and sustain.
- Keeping your hips forward, toes to the ceiling, raise your leg up as far as your flexibility will allow and return to the starting position.
- Repeat on other side.
- Try this exercise with the toe pointing both down and up to target different muscle groups.
- Strengthens buttocks, thighs and core.

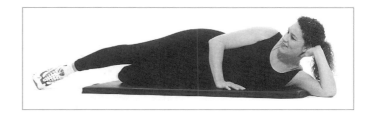

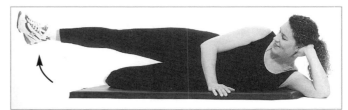

Sidelying leg lifts.

Alternating Standing Lunges

- Stand with your feet together and arms at your sides, holding dumbbells.
- Fire the core and sustain.
- Keeping your back straight and your head up, take a large step forward.
- Bend until your front thigh is parallel to the floor, ensuring that at the bottom of the movement your front knee does not pass your toes. Your back leg should be almost straight and should not touch the floor.
- Always exhale on exertion.
- Strengthens buttocks, thighs and core.

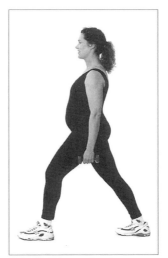
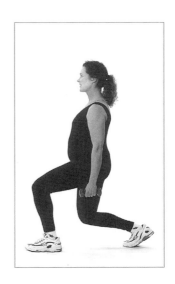

Alternating standing lunges.

Front Step-ups

- Stand facing a stool or step, keeping your shoulders back as you fire the core and sustain.
- Holding a dumbbell in each hand, exhale as you step up onto the stool.
- This exercise can be done with or without weights.
- Ensure that the stool you are stepping onto is not placing your knee beyond 90 degrees.
- Strengthens buttocks, thighs and core.

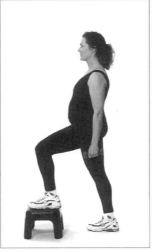
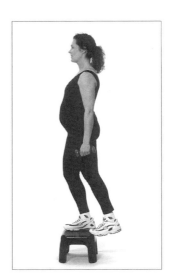

Front step-ups.

Sample Strength Workouts with Weights

What Is Your Fitness Level?

The Fit to Deliver program is designed so it can be used by beginning and experienced exercisers alike. In order to get the most out of this program, start by answering the following questions.

What trimester are you in?

Trimester 1   0 to 12 weeks
Trimester 2   13 to 27 weeks
Trimester 3   28 weeks to delivery

What was your pre-pregnancy fitness level?

Fitness level prior to beginning an exercise program or class

A. Beginner
  • I have never worked out before; or
  • I have not exercised consistently (minimum three times per week) for at least three months; or
  • I have little to no experience with strength or resistance training.

B. Intermediate
  • I work out consistently three to five times per week; or
  • I am active in sports; and
  • I include cardiovascular, strength and flexibility training in my program.

C. Advanced
  • I work out consistently five or more days per week;
  • I have an athletic background;
  • I have been working out at least six months prior to pregnancy.

Warm-up Program

Suggested warm-ups differ by trimester, because higher impact activities, such as jogging, skipping and butt kicks, may become less comfortable as pregnancy progresses. If an exercise becomes uncomfortable substitute it with another (for example, walking for jogging). Remember to stay well hydrated, and don't overheat or become overly fatigued.

Dynamic Warm-up #1 (first trimester)

Walk, jog or skip for 7–10 minutes, then do some general light jogging drills such as skips, butt kicks, side shuffles, crossover runs and high knees over a distance of 10–20 meters. Progress to dynamic flexibility exercises such as leg swings front and back, side to side and in a figure-8 pattern. Torso twists, arm swings and mini lunges also help with an overall warm-up.

Trimester 1—Beginner

Current guidelines suggest that all women get moving and reap the benefits of exercise. This includes women in the first trimester of their pregnancy. If you did not exercise be-

TIPS FROM THE TEAM

• Be flexible. As your body changes, modify your program.
• Decrease the weight, decrease sets and decrease reps if needed.
• Increase your recovery time between sets or between exercise sessions.
• Exhale as you perform the work portion of the exercise and inhale as you relax.
• Never hold your breath (Valsalva maneuver) while lifting.

fore pregnancy consult your physician prior to starting, then begin a moderate exercise program like the one outlined below.

These exercises are not exhaustive and you may add others from the book based on your experience or on the advice of your healthcare or fitness professional.

Warm-up

You can do the general dynamic warm-up.

Walking Routine (see page 61 for suggested workouts)

Begin with 10–15 minutes in one exercise session. You should do this for a week before increasing the duration. Walking can be done every day if you feel up to it.

Gradually increase the time each week. By your twelfth week you should be able to walk for a full 30 minutes while still being able to perform the talk test or staying

within the Rate of Perceived Exertion guidelines of 3–5.

Pregnancy is not the time to make great fitness gains. Rather, the first twelve weeks will help you prepare for the aerobic and strength exercises that you will be able to perform once you are in your second trimester.

> *All exercise descriptions can be found in this chapter or in chapter 3, The Core.*

Core (Trunk) and Pelvic Floor Stability

Choose 2–4 exercises, and change them regularly. Add some of your favorite exercises that strengthen the core as well as other muscles.

- Five on the Floor, including Tighten (Fire the Core and Sustain) with Leg Slide, Leg Fall Out (abduction), March, and Dying Bug
- 4-Point Kneeling Pony Back to Neutral (suck in your tummy and round your back)
- Supine Bridging (stomach up)
- Supine Bridging (with stretch cord abduction)
- Clamshell
- Circus Ponies (alternating arm and leg raises; use ball or on all fours)

Choose 2 exercises
- Kegel Exercises, including Hold-ems, Speed-ems, Squeeze-ems and Elevate-ems
- Belly Button Breaths (in through nose, out through mouth HA HA HA)
- Baby Hugs (big, bigger, biggest)

TIPS FROM THE TEAM

- Include "crazy walks" in your cooldown program to strengthen the muscles of the lower leg and foot. Try walking for five meters on your heels to strengthen the lower leg muscles.
- Walking backward helps to stretch out the hip flexors in the front of the thigh.

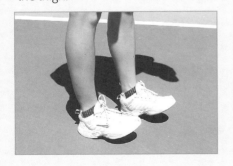

Cooldown and Stretching

Have another drink of water and evaluate how you feel. You can now do light stretching exercises as described in chapter 5.

Trimester 1—Intermediate

Warm-up

- 15 minutes on an exercise bike or walking on a treadmill.
- Rate of Perceived Exertion: 3–5, or use the talk test.
- Do Dynamic Warm-up exercises (see chapter 5).

Upper Body

- Do 1–2 sets of 10–15 repetitions.
- Choose 2 exercises for back and 1 exercise for all other muscle groups, and change them regularly.

Back

- Bent Over One-Arm Rows (weight or cord for resistance)
- Standing Row (pulley or cord)
- Seated Row
- Lat Pulldowns (wide grip) overhand (not shown)
- Lat Pulldowns (narrow grip) underhand (not shown)

Chest

- Seated Chest Press (weight or cord for resistance)
- Incline Bench Press (with or without stool)
- Flat Bench Press (not shown)
- Incline Flys (weight for resistance)
- Wall Push-ups or Push-ups (with bent knees, or on toes)

Shoulders

- Lateral Raises, standing or seated
- Bent Over Lateral Raises
- Front Shoulder Raises, standing or seated
- Standing Two-Arm Row
- Lateral (external) Rotation
- Medial (internal) Rotation

Triceps

- Tricep Kickbacks
- Tricep Flatbar Press
- Tricep Incline Press (not shown)
- Dips (hands on a chair, with knees bent or straight legs) (not shown)
- Standing Push-ups (with hands close together)

Biceps

- Bicep Dumbbell Curls
- Bicep Pulley Curls

Lower Body

- Do 1–3 sets of 15–20 repetitions.
- Choose 2 exercises for each muscle group, and change them regularly.

Front Thigh and Inner Thigh

- Squats on the wall (use ball)
- Resisted Squats (use stretch cord for resistance)
- Dumbbell 1/3 Squats
- Front Step-ups
- Split Squats
- Sidelying Adduction

Back Thigh and Outer Thigh

- Side Step-ups
- Sidelying Abduction (leg lift)
- Standing Hip Abductions (use cord for resistance)

- Alternating Standing Lunges
- Seated Hamstring Cable Curls

Core (Trunk) and Pelvic Floor Stability

Choose 2–4 exercises, and change them regularly. Add some of your favorite exercises that strengthen the core as well as other muscles.

- Five on the Floor, including Tighten (Fire the Core and Sustain) with Leg Slide, Leg Fall Out (abduction), March and Dying Bug
- 4-Point Kneeling Pony Back to Neutral (suck in your tummy and round your back)
- Supine Bridging (stomach up)
- Supine Bridging (with stretch cord abduction)
- Clamshell
- Circus Ponies (alternating arm and leg raises; use ball or on all fours)

Choose 2 exercises
- Kegel Exercises, including Hold-ems, Speed-ems, Squeeze-ems and Elevate-ems
- Belly Button Breaths (in through nose, out through mouth HA HA HA)
- Baby Hugs (big, bigger, biggest)

To effectively fire the core and sustain you must follow these principles:
- Ensure that the initial contraction is isolated (no other muscles substituting).
- The contraction should begin slowly with control.
- Low effort is all that is required.
- Breathe normally.

Cooldown and Stretching
- Evaluate how you feel. Have a drink of water.
- Concentrate on stretching the pectorals, hamstrings, low back and hip flexors.

Trimester 1—Advanced
Warm-up
- 15 minutes on an exercise bike or walking on a treadmill.
- Rate of Perceived Exertion: 3–5, or use the talk test.
- Do Dynamic Warm-up exercises (see chapter 5).

Upper Body
- Do 2–3 sets of 10–15 repetitions.
- Choose 2 exercises for back and 1–2 exercises for all other muscle groups, and change them regularly.

Back
- Bent Over One-Arm Rows
- Standing Row
- Seated Row
- Lat Pulldowns (wide grip) overhand (not shown)
- Lat Pulldowns (narrow grip) underhand (not shown)

Chest
- Seated Chest Press (weight or cord for resistance)
- Incline Bench Press (with or without stool)
- Flat Bench Press (not shown)
- Incline Flys (weight for resistance)
- Wall Push-ups or Push-ups (with bent knees, or on toes)

Shoulders

- Lateral Raises, standing or seated
- Bent Over Lateral Raises
- Front Shoulder Raises, standing or seated
- Standing Two-Arm Row
- Lateral (external) Rotation
- Medial (internal) Rotation

Triceps

- Tricep Kickbacks
- Tricep Flatbar Press
- Tricep Incline Press
- Dips (hands on a chair, with knees bent, or straight legs) (not shown)
- Standing Push-ups (with hands close together)

Biceps

- Bicep Dumbbell Curls
- Bicep Pulley Curls

Lower Body

- Do 1–3 sets of 15–20 repetitions.
- Choose 2 exercises for each muscle group, and change them regularly.

Front Thigh and Inner Thigh

- Squats on the wall (use ball)
- Dumbbell 1/3 Squats
- Front Step-ups
- Split Squats
- Sidelying Adduction

Back Thigh and Outer Thigh

- Side Step-ups
- Sidelying Abduction (leg lift)
- Standing Hip Abductions (use cord for resistance)
- Alternating Standing Lunges
- Seated Hamstring Cable Curls

Core (Trunk) and Pelvic Floor Stability

Choose 2–4 exercises, and change them regularly. Add some of your favorite exercises that strengthen the core as well as other muscles.

- Five on the Floor, including Tighten (Fire the Core and Sustain) with Leg Slide, Leg Fall Out (abduction), March and Dying Bug
- Pony Back to Neutral (suck in your tummy and round your back)
- Supine Bridging (stomach up)
- Supine Bridging (with stretch cord abduction)
- Clamshell
- Circus Ponies (alternating arm and leg raises; use ball or on all fours)

Choose 2 exercises

- Kegel Exercises, including Hold-ems, Speed-ems, Squeeze-ems and Elevate-ems
- Belly Button Breaths (in through nose, out through mouth HA HA HA)
- Baby Hugs (big, bigger, biggest)

To effectively fire the core and sustain you must follow these principles:

- Ensure that the initial contraction is isolated (no other muscles substituting).
- The contraction should begin slowly with control.
- Low effort is all that is required.
- Breathe normally.

Cooldown and Stretching

- Evaluate how you feel. Have a drink of water.
- Concentrate on stretching the pectorals, hamstrings, low back and hip flexors.

Dynamic Warm-up #2 (second trimester)

Walk, easy jog or ride a stationary bicycle or swim for 5–10 minutes, then do some general loosening exercises in the gym. These can include dynamic hip flexibility exercises such as leg swings front and back, side to side and in a figure-8 pattern. Torso twists, arm swings and mini lunges also help with an overall warm-up.

Dynamic Warm-up #3 (third trimester)

Walk or ride a stationary bicycle or swim for 5–10 minutes, then do some general loosening exercises either in the gym or in the shallow end of the pool. These can include dynamic hip flexibility exercises such as leg swings front and back, side to side and in a figure-8 motion. Torso twists, arm swings and shoulder shrugs also help with an overall warm-up. Hang onto a wall or fence when doing leg swings to aid balance and ensure a full range of motion.

Trimesters 2 & 3—Beginner

Warm-up

- 15 minutes on an exercise bike or walking on a treadmill.
- Rate of Perceived Exertion: 3–5, or use the talk test.
- Do Dynamic Warm-up exercises (see chapter 5).

Upper Body

- Do 1–2 sets of 10–15 repetitions.
- Choose 2 exercises for back and 1 exercise for all other muscle groups, and change them regularly.

Back

- Bent Over One-Arm Rows
- Standing Row
- Seated Row
- Lat Pulldowns (wide grip) overhand (not shown)
- Lat Pulldowns (narrow grip) underhand (not shown)

Chest

- Seated Chest Press (weight or cord for resistance)
- Incline Bench Press (with or without stool)
- Flat Bench Press (not shown)
- Incline Flys (weight for resistance)
- Wall Push-ups or Push-ups (with bent knees, or on toes)

Shoulders

- Lateral Raises, standing or seated
- Bent Over Lateral Raises
- Front Shoulder Raises, standing or seated
- Standing Two-Arm Row
- Lateral (external) Rotation
- Medial (internal) Rotation

Triceps

- Tricep Kickbacks
- Tricep Flatbar Press
- Tricep Incline Press
- Dips (hands on a chair, with knees bent, or straight legs) (not shown)
- Wall Push-ups (with hands close together) (not shown)

Biceps

- Bicep Dumbbell Curls
- Bicep Pulley Curls

Lower Body

- Do 1–3 sets of 15–20 repetitions.
- Choose 2 exercises for each muscle group, and change them regularly.

Front Thigh and Inner Thigh

- Squats on the wall (use ball)
- Dumbbell 1/3 Squats
- Front Step-ups
- Split Squats
- Sidelying Adduction

Back Thigh and Outer Thigh

- Side Step-ups
- Sidelying Abduction (leg lift)
- Standing Hip Abductions (use cord for resistance)
- Alternating Standing Lunges
- Seated Hamstring Cable Curls

Core (Trunk) and Pelvic Floor Stability

- Choose 2–4 exercises, and change them regularly. Add some of your favorite exercises that strengthen the core as well as other muscles.
- Five on the Floor, including Tighten (Fire the Core and Sustain) with Leg Slide, Leg Fall Out (abduction), March and Dying Bug
- Pony Back to Neutral (suck in your tummy and round your back)
- Supine Bridging (stomach up)

> **NOTE**
>
> *Supine bridging exercises that last more than 30 seconds can be done in the first trimester. During the second and third trimesters you can exercise for 30 seconds, then roll to your left side for a rest before continuing.*

- Supine Bridging (with stretch cord abduction)
- Clamshell
- Circus Ponies (alternating arm and leg raises; use ball or on all fours)

Choose 2 exercises
- Kegel Exercises, including Hold-ems, Speed-ems, Squeeze-ems and Elevate-ems
- Baby Hugs (big, bigger, biggest)
- Belly Button Breaths (in through nose, out through mouth HA HA HA)

To effectively fire the core and sustain you must follow these principles:
- Ensure that the initial contraction is isolated (no other muscles substituting).
- The contraction should begin slowly with control.
- Low effort is all that is required.
- Breathe normally.

Cooldown and Stretching

- Evaluate how you feel. Have a drink of water.
- Concentrate on stretching the pectorals, hamstrings, low back and hip flexors.

Trimesters 2 & 3—Intermediate
Warm-up

- 15 minutes on an exercise bike or walking on a treadmill.
- Rate of Perceived Exertion: 3–5, or use the talk test.
- Do Dynamic Warm-up exercises (see chapter 5).

Upper Body

- Do 2–3 sets of 10–15 repetitions.
- Choose 2 exercises for back and 1–2 exer-

cises for all other muscle groups, and change them regularly.

Back
- Bent Over One-Arm Rows
- Standing Row
- Seated Row
- Lat Pulldowns (wide grip) overhand (not shown)
- Lat Pulldowns (narrow grip) underhand (not shown)

Chest
- Seated Chest Press (weight or cord for resistance)
- Incline Bench Press (with or without stool)
- Flat Bench Press (not shown)
- Incline Flys (weight for resistance)
- Wall Push-ups or Push-ups (with bent knees, or on toes)

Shoulders
- Lateral Raises, standing or seated
- Bent Over Lateral Raises
- Front Shoulder Raises, standing or seated
- Standing Two-Arm Row
- Lateral (external) Rotation
- Medial (internal) Rotation

Triceps
- Tricep Kickbacks
- Tricep Flatbar Press
- Tricep Incline Press
- Dips (hands on a chair, with knees bent, or straight legs) (not shown)
- Standing Push-ups (with hands close together) (not shown)

Biceps
- Bicep Dumbbell Curls
- Bicep Pulley Curls

Lower Body
- Do 2–3 sets of 15–20 repetitions.
- Choose 2 exercises for each muscle group, and change them regularly.

Front Thigh and Inner Thigh
- Squats on the wall (use ball)
- Dumbbell 1/3 Squats
- Front Step-ups
- Split Squats
- Sidelying Adduction

Back Thigh and Outer Thigh
- Side Step-ups
- Sidelying Abduction (leg lift)
- Standing Hip Abductions (use cord for resistance)
- Alternating Standing Lunges
- Seated Hamstring Cable Curls

Core (Trunk) and Pelvic Floor Stability
Choose 2–4 exercises, and change them regularly. Add some of your favorite exercises that strengthen the core as well as other muscles.
- Five on the Floor, including Tighten (Fire the Core and Sustain) with Leg Slide, Leg Fall Out (abduction), March and Dying Bug
- Pony Back to Neutral (suck in your tummy and round your back)
- Supine Bridging (stomach up)

> **NOTE**
> *Supine bridging exercises that last more than 30 seconds can be done in the first trimester. During the second and third trimesters you can exercise for 30 seconds, then roll to your left side for a rest before continuing.*

- Supine Bridging (with stretch cord abduction)
- Clamshell
- Circus Ponies (alternating arm and leg raises; use ball or on all fours)

Choose 2 exercises
- Kegel Exercises, including Hold-ems, Speed-ems, Squeeze-ems and Elevate-ems
- Belly Button Breaths (in through nose, out through mouth HA HA HA)
- Baby Hugs (big, bigger, biggest)

To effectively fire the core and sustain you must follow these principles:
- Ensure that the initial contraction is isolated (no other muscles substituting).
- The contraction should begin slowly with control.
- Low effort is all that is required.
- Breathe normally.

Cooldown and Stretching
- Evaluate how you feel. Have a drink of water.
- Concentrate on stretching the pectorals, hamstrings, low back and hip flexors.

Trimesters 2 & 3—Advanced
Warm-up
- 15 minutes on an exercise bike or walking on a treadmill.
- Rate of Perceived Exertion: 3–5, or use the talk test.
- Do Dynamic Warm-up exercises (see chapter 5).

Upper Body
- Do 2–3 sets of 10–15 repetitions.
- Choose 2 exercises for back and 2 exercises for all other muscle groups, and change them regularly.

Back
- Bent Over One-Arm Rows
- Standing Row
- Seated Row
- Lat Pulldowns (wide grip) overhand (not shown)
- Lat Pulldowns (narrow grip) underhand (not shown)

Chest
- Seated Chest Press (weight or cord for resistance)
- Incline Bench Press (with or without stool)
- Flat Bench Press (not shown)
- Incline Flys (weight for resistance)
- Wall Push-ups or Push-ups (with bent knees, or on toes)

Shoulders
- Lateral Raises, standing or seated
- Bent Over Lateral Raises
- Front Shoulder Raises, standing or seated
- Standing Two-Arm Row
- Lateral (external) Rotation
- Medial (internal) Rotation

Triceps
- Tricep Kickbacks
- Tricep Flatbar Press
- Tricep Incline Press
- Dips (hands on a chair, with knees bent, or straight legs) (not shown)
- Standing Push-ups (with hands close together) (not shown)

Biceps
- Bicep Dumbbell Curls
- Bicep Pulley Curls

Lower Body
- Do 2–3 sets of 15–20 repetitions.
- Choose 2 exercises for each muscle group, and change them regularly.

Front Thigh and Inner Thigh
- Squats on the wall (use ball)
- Dumbbell 1/3 Squats
- Front Step-ups
- Split Squats
- Sidelying Adduction

Back Thigh and Outer Thigh
- Side Step-ups
- Sidelying Abduction (leg lift)
- Standing Hip Abductions (use cord for resistance)
- Alternating Standing Lunges
- Seated Hamstring Cable Curls

Core (Trunk) and Pelvic Floor Stability

Choose 2–4 exercises, and change them regularly. Add some of your favorite exercises that strengthen the core as well as other muscles.
- Five on the Floor, including Tighten (Fire the Core and Sustain) with Leg Slide, Leg Fall Out (abduction), March and Dying Bug
- Pony Back to Neutral (suck in your tummy and round your back)
- Supine Bridging (stomach up)
- Supine Bridging (with stretch cord abduction)
- Clamshell

- Circus Ponies (alternating arm and leg raises; use ball or on all fours)

Choose 2 exercises
- Kegel Exercises, including Hold-ems, Speed-ems, Squeeze-ems and Elevate-ems
- Belly Button Breaths (in through nose, out through mouth HA HA HA)
- Baby Hugs (big, bigger, biggest)

To effectively fire the core and sustain you must follow these principles:
- Ensure that the initial contraction is isolated (no other muscles substituting).
- The contraction should begin slowly with control.
- Low effort is all that is required.
- Breathe normally.

Cooldown and Stretching
- Evaluate how you feel. Have a drink of water.
- Concentrate on stretching the pectorals, hamstrings, low back and hip flexors.

NOTE

Supine bridging exercises that last more than 30 seconds can be done in the first trimester. During the second and third trimesters you can exercise for 30 seconds, then roll to your left side for a rest before continuing.

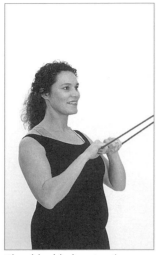
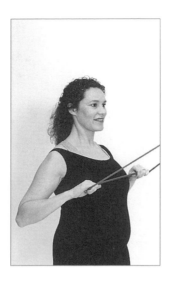

Shoulder blade retraction.

Stretch Cord Workouts
Upper Body
Shoulder Blade Retraction

- Stand with your core fired and sustain, knees slightly bent.
- Pull the cord down to your chest and then apart, concentrating on using the muscles in your back and shoulders.

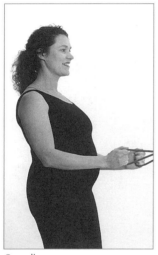
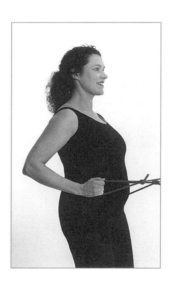

Standing two-arm row.

Standing Two-Arm Row

- Stand with your core fired and sustain, knees slightly bent and shoulders square.
- Keep your shoulders down, and exhale as you bring your elbows back until your wrists meet your hips.

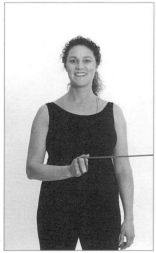
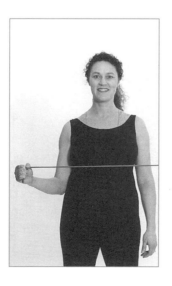

Lateral rotation.

Lateral Rotation

- Stand with your core fired and sustain, keeping shoulders square.
- Keep your elbows at your side for the entire exercise.
- Exhale as you bring your arm away from your body.

Medial Rotation

- Stand with your core fired and sustain, keeping shoulders square.
- Keep your elbows at your side for the entire exercise.
- Exhale as you bring your arm toward your body.

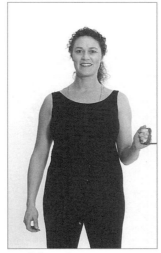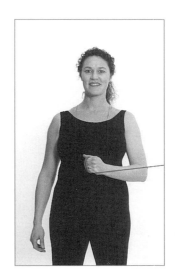

Medial rotation.

Standing Push-up

- This exercise can be done on any wall, countertop, doorframe or stable object.
- Keep your core fired and sustain and shoulders square, hands shoulder-width apart.
- Gently lower yourself toward the wall, maintaining good posture.
- Exhale as you return to your starting position.

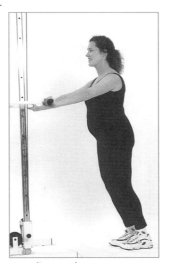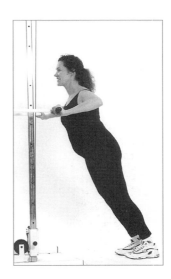

Standing push-up.

Lower Body

Do 1–3 sets of 15–20 repetitions.

Cross-Country Extension

- Place the theraband under your foot.
- Fire the core and sustain, keeping shoulders square.
- Start with your knee up, holding onto a chair for support.
- Exhale as you extend your leg behind you, being sure not to arch your back.

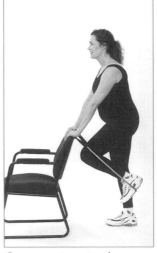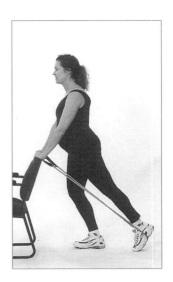

Cross-country extension.

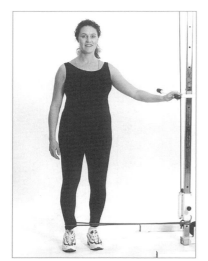 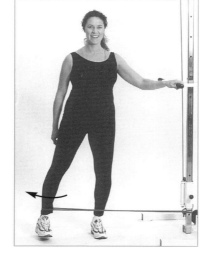 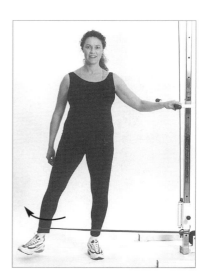

Standing hip abductions.

Standing Hip Abductions

- Start with very light resistance.
- Stand tall with your core fired and sustain and knee slightly bent (soft) on supporting leg.
- Hold onto something stable, such as a chair or table, for balance.
- With your toe pointing in and/or out exhale as you lift your leg out to the side.

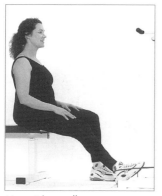 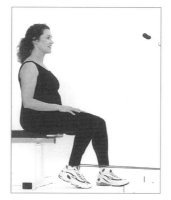

Hamstring pulls.

Hamstring Pulls

- This exercise can be done with a cable or a theraband.
- Sit tall on a bench, keeping your core fired and sustain.
- Keep your foot slightly off the floor.
- Exhale as you draw your heel toward you.

Band Mini Squats

- With your feet hip-width apart place a theraband around your legs, just above your knees.
- Hold a dumbbell in each hand.
- Fire the core and sustain.
- Exhale as you slowly lower your torso while pressing your knees to the outside of your foot.
- To perform this exercise without weights, just place your hands on your hips.

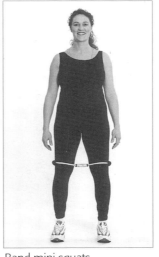 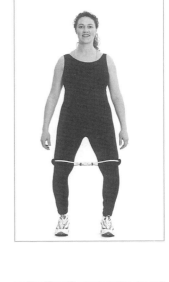

Band mini squats.

Resisted Squats

- Step onto a stretch cord with both feet, hip-width apart.
- Fire the core and sustain.
- Hold one handle in each hand with your knees bent, and exhale as you stand up. Always keep knees slightly bent.

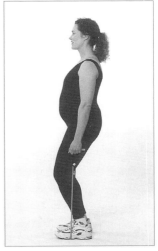 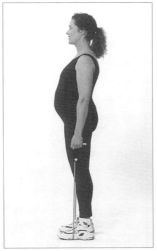

Resisted squats.

Step-ups with Cord Pull

- Stand facing a stool, fire the core and sustain and shoulders back.
- Hold a stretch cord that is attached above.
- Exhale as you step up onto a stool and pull the cord down.
- Ensure that the stool you are stepping onto is not placing your knee beyond 90 degrees.

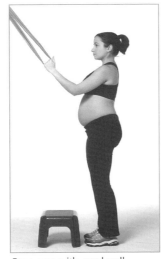 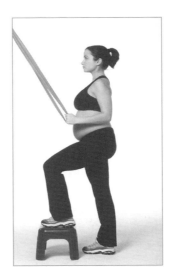 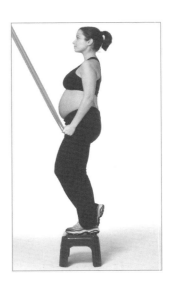

Step-ups with cord pull.

Core (Trunk) and Pelvic Floor Stability

Follow the exercises listed appropriate to your trimester in the Strength Training workouts.

Sample Stretch Cord/Home Workouts

Trimester 1

Warm-up

- 15 minutes on an exercise bike or walking on a treadmill.
- Rate of Perceived Exertion: 3–5, or use the talk test.
- Do Dynamic Warm-up exercises (see chapter 5).

Upper Body

- Do 1–3 sets of 10–15 repetitions.
- Choose 2 exercises for back and 1–2 exercises for all other muscle groups, and change them regularly.

NOTE *All exercise descriptions are found in this chapter.*

TIPS FROM THE TEAM

- Avoid doing resisted inner thigh (adductor) or hip flexor strength exercises because the muscles tend to naturally shorten and stiffen as pregnancy progresses.
- Avoid being on your back for prolonged periods of time (more than 30 seconds) after the first trimester.

Back

- Bent Over One-Arm Rows (weight or cord for resistance)
- Standing Row (use cord for resistance)
- Seated Row (use cord for resistance) (not shown)
- Lat Cord Pulldowns
- Straight Arm Cord Pulldowns

Chest

- Standing or Seated Chest Press (cord for resistance)
- Incline Bench Press (weight or light cord for resistance)
- Flat Bench Press (not shown)
- Incline Flys (weight for resistance)
- Push-ups (with bent knees, or on toes)

Shoulders

- Shoulder Blade Retractions (use cord for resistance)
- Lateral Raises, standing or seated
- Bent Over Lateral Raises
- Front Shoulder Raises, standing or seated (light cord resistance)
- Standing Two-Arm Row
- Lateral (external) Rotation with stretch cord
- Medial (internal) Rotation with stretch cord

Triceps

- Tricep Kickbacks (weight or light cord for resistance)
- Tricep Cord Press
- Tricep Incline Press
- Wall Push-ups (with hands close together)

Biceps

- Bicep Cord Curls (standing or seated, single arm or together)
- Bicep Curls (light weights or cans; can also be done with arms externally rotated)

Lower Body

- Do 1–3 sets of 15–20 repetitions.
- Choose 2 exercises for each muscle group, and change them regularly.

Front Thigh and Inner Thigh

- Squats on the wall (use ball)
- Resisted Squats (use stretch cord for resistance)
- Dumbbell 1/3 Squats
- Front Step-ups with Cord Pull
- Sidelying Adduction

Back Thigh and Outer Thigh

- Cross Country Extension
- Side Step-ups
- Sidelying Abduction (leg lift)
- Standing Hip Abductions (use cord for resistance)
- Alternating Standing Lunges
- Standing Hamstring Curl
- Seated Hamstring Cord Curls

Core (Trunk) and Pelvic Floor Stability

Choose 2–4 exercises, and change them regularly. Add some of your favorite exercises that strengthen the core as well as other muscles.

- Five on the Floor, including Tighten (Fire the Core and Sustain) with Leg Slide, Leg Fall Out (abduction), March and Dying Bug

- Pony Back to Neutral (suck in your tummy and round your back)
- Supine Bridging (stomach up)
- Supine Bridging (with stretch cord abduction)
- Clamshell
- Circus Ponies (alternating arm and leg raises; use ball or on all fours)

Choose 2 exercises

- Kegel Exercises, including Hold-ems, Speed-ems, Squeeze-ems and Elevate-ems
- Belly Button Breaths (in through nose, out through mouth HA HA HA)
- Baby Hugs (big, bigger, biggest)

Cooldown and Stretching

- Evaluate how you feel. Have a drink of water.
- Concentrate on stretching the pectorals, hamstrings, low back and hip flexors.

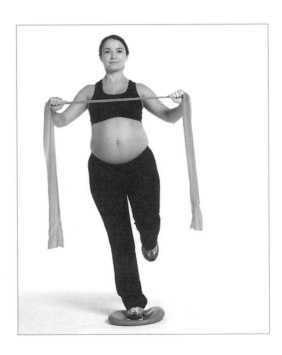

Trimesters 2 & 3

Warm-up

- 15 minutes on an exercise bike or walking on a treadmill.
- Rate of Perceived Exertion: 3–5, or use the talk test.
- Do Dynamic Warm-up exercises (see chapter 5).

Upper Body

- Do 1–3 sets of 10–15 repetitions.
- Choose 2 exercises for back and 1 exercise for all other muscle groups, and change them regularly.

Back

- Bent Over One-Arm Rows (weight or cord for resistance)
- Standing Row (use cord for resistance)
- Seated Row (use cord for resistance) (not shown)
- Lat Cord Pulldowns
- Straight Arm Cord Pulldowns

Chest

- Standing or Seated Chest Press (cord for resistance)
- Incline Bench Press (weight or light cord for resistance)
- Incline Flys (weight for resistance)
- Push-ups (with bent knees, or on toes)

Shoulders

- Shoulder Blade Retractions (use cord for resistance)
- Lateral Raises, standing or seated
- Bent Over Lateral Raises
- Front Shoulder Raises, standing or seated (light cord resistance)
- Standing Two-Arm Row

- Bicep Curl and Lateral Raise
- Lateral (external) Rotation
- Medial (internal) Rotation

Triceps

- Tricep Kickbacks (weight or light cord for resistance)
- Tricep Cord Press
- Tricep Incline Press
- Dips (hands on a chair, with knees bent)
- Wall Push-ups (with hands close together)

Biceps

- Bicep Cord Curls (standing or seated, single arm or together)
- Bicep Curls (light weights or cans; can also be done with arms externally rotated)

Lower Body

- Do 1–3 sets of 15–20 repetitions.
- Choose 2 exercises for each muscle group, and change them regularly.

Front Thigh and Inner Thigh

- Squats on the wall (use ball)
- Resisted Squats
- Dumbbell 1/3 Squats
- Front Step-ups with Cord Pull
- Sidelying Adduction

Back Thigh and Outer Thigh

- Cross Country Extension
- Side Step-ups
- Sidelying Abduction (leg lift)
- Standing Hip Abductions (use cord for resistance)
- Alternating Standing Lunges
- Standing Hamstring Curl
- Seated Hamstring Cord Curls

Core (Trunk) and Pelvic Floor Stability

Choose 2–4 exercises, and change them regularly. Add some of your favorite exercises that strengthen the core as well as other muscles.

- Five on the Floor, including Tighten (Fire the Core and Sustain) with Leg Slide, Leg Fall Out (abduction), March and Dying Bug
- Pony Back to Neutral (suck in your tummy and round your back)
- Supine Bridging (stomach up)
- Supine Bridging (with stretch cord abduction)
- Sidelying Knee-ups
- Clamshell
- Circus Ponies (alternating arm and leg raises; on all fours)

Choose 2 exercises
- Kegel Exercises, including Hold-ems, Speed-ems, Squeeze-ems and Elevate-ems
- Belly Button Breaths (in through nose, out through mouth HA HA HA)
- Baby Hugs (big, bigger, biggest)

> **NOTE**
>
> *Supine bridging exercises that last more than 30 seconds can be done in the first trimester. During the second and third trimesters you can exercise for 30 seconds, then roll to your left side for a rest before continuing.*

Cooldown and Stretching

- Evaluate how you feel. Have a drink of water.
- Concentrate on stretching the pectorals, hamstrings, low back and hip flexors.

To effectively fire the core and sustain you must follow these principles:
- Ensure that the initial contraction is isolated (no other muscles substituting).
- The contraction should begin slowly with control.
- Low effort is all that is required.
- Breathe normally.

> **TIPS FROM THE TEAM**
>
> **Post-Exercise Recovery Techniques**
> - Avoid saunas and whirlpools, due to concerns about an increase in core body temperature.
> - Using warmth and cold will help aid recovery, but avoid placing ice directly over the abdomen or sacrum (base of spine). Be sure to get direction from your physical therapist or physician.
> - After an appropriate cooldown, relaxation exercises can be included. See chapter 9 for ideas.

8

Balance Training

Balance training is a fundamental component of daily life and should be a part of everyone's fitness routine. During pregnancy and the postpartum period the hormonal, physical and postural changes that occur make it extremely important to continue training balance to keep you stable. Improving balance will allow you to perform daily activities easily and safely, and will improve your confidence with new activities or sports. Your body will be able to react to unexpected events and protect itself during repetitive motions.

General Benefits

- Improves balance, coordination, timing and agility.
- Fires the core automatically.
- Improves joint proprioception.
- Improves stability in the joints of the ankle, knee, hip and spine.
- Helps prevent repetitive strain injuries.
- Helps prevent falls and injuries.
- Motivates you to train and is fun.

Balance reactions can be trained simply by doing single leg stance and leg swing activities that you use as part of your dynamic warm-up. You may want to hold on to a chair for added stability.

Add a balance component to normal exercises by providing an unstable base like an exercise ball, wobble board, Sissel disc, ½ foam roll or balance machine like the dynamic edge, pro fitter or Reebok core board.

Rolled Towel, Wobble Board, ½ Foam Roll or Sissel Disc Exercises

- A rolled towel, wobble board, ½ foam roll or Sissel disc can be incorporated into many basic exercises to add a balance challenge.
- Start by standing with one foot on a rolled

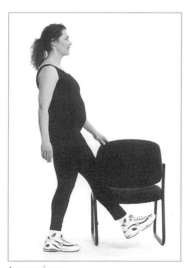

Leg swings.

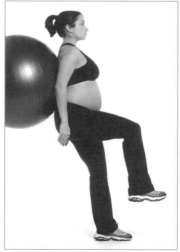

Exercise ball balance.

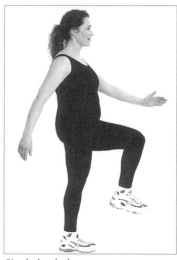

Single leg balance.

towel, ½ foam roll or Sissel disc, or stand with both feet on a wobble board. You can make the exercise more challenging by holding light dumbbells or using a thera-band to do some resistance work at the same time.

- Keep a soft bend in your supporting knee.
- Try doing 10 alternating bicep curls to begin.
- When you are comfortable with bicep curls you can try front or lateral shoulder raises, hammer curls or cord pulls, etc.
- Remember to fire the core and sustain throughout the exercise.
- This exercise can be changed to hip abduction (raise leg out to the side), with one leg on the Sissel disk.

Exercise Ball Balance

Just sitting on an exercise ball can be a challenge as your pregnancy progresses. Do some torso rotatations or lift one leg to further improve your balance.

Training Tips

- Before or during each training session, be sure to perform some exercises that focus on balance.
- Elastic tubing can be used with all balance equipment to add an upper body or extra core component to training.

> **NOTE**
> These exercises are not exhaustive and you may add others based on your experience or on the advice of your healthcare or fitness professional.

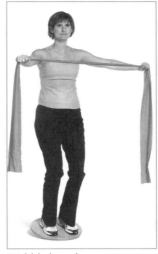

Wobble board.

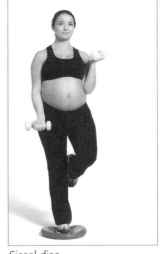

Sissel disc.

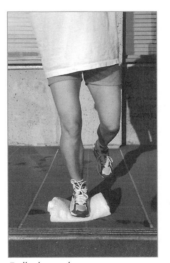

Rolled towel.

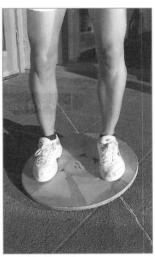

Wobble board.

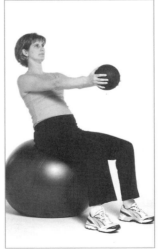
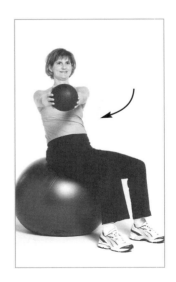

Exercise ball balance.

Exercise Ball and Band Workouts
Three-Dimensional Training

Traditional strength exercises and aerobic equipment often constrain us to a single plane of movement. For example, exercises like bicep curls involve a single joint and are in one plane of movement. Machines such as the treadmill, stationary bike and stair-climber also work the body in only one plane of movement. Real life is three-dimensional and our bodies are constantly challenged to react dynamically to the moving, changing environment in which we live and play. Activity requires strength and coordination in three planes of movement.

You will find that 3-D training with an exercise ball will help improve balance and body awareness. By training on its unstable surface your balance reactions and coordination are working subconsciously, helping them to become automatic. This helps to prevent injury and improve your ability to carry out the activities of daily living including sports.

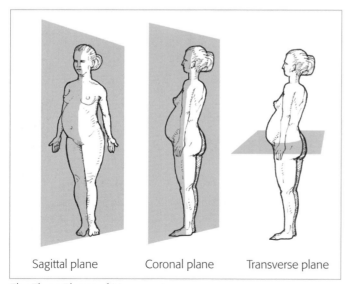

Sagittal plane   Coronal plane   Transverse plane

The Three Planes of Movement.

Ball Precautions
- Avoid placing the ball near heat or in direct sunlight.
- Avoid sharp objects and jewellery.
- Start gradually and get a feel for the ball before progressing.
- If you are new to exercise, check with your physician before you begin any fitness program.

Before You Start

Choosing the proper ball size is important. When you sit on the ball, your knees should be bent to 90 degrees with your feet flat on the floor. The hips should be bent to almost 90 degrees but should be resting equal to or slightly higher than the height of your knees.

The following exercises are designed to help to develop the core and to strengthen specific larger muscles in a dynamic and functional way. Before getting started perform the warm-up exercises outlined in chapter 5, and when you are finished cool down with the exercises in chapter 5.

Fire the Core and Sustain

Before each exercise focus on the following:
- Contract the pelvic floor (Kegel).
- Contract the TA (lower abdominal).
- Remember to breathe.
- Keep knees soft if standing.

For each of the following exercises, perform 2–3 sets of 10–15 repetitions unless otherwise specified.

Ball Sitting Dead Bugs
- Sit in the middle of the ball with feet flat on the floor, shoulder-width apart.
- Fire the core and sustain.

- Raise arms out to the side to 90 degrees with elbows bent.
- Bring right elbow across your body to meet the left knee in the middle. Keep your core muscles tightened throughout the exercise. Start by doing 2 sets of 15 repetitions, then increase as you are able.
- Strengthens core.

Ball Bridges

(After the first trimester, lie on your back for only 30 seconds at a time.)

- Lie on your back on a mat with your feet on the ball.
- Keep the head and arms relaxed.
- Fire the core and sustain, and don't grip with your buttocks.
- Lift your hips and low back (from tailbone to ribcage) until trunk is level with thighs.
- Weight should be on the upper back, not the neck.
- Keep your spine neutral.
- Strengthens core, lower back and buttocks.

Wall Ball Squats

- Place an exercise ball at your mid back against the wall.
- Fire the core and sustain, and place feet shoulder-width apart.
- Start with 2 sets of 10 repetitions, and increase to 3 sets of 20 repetitions. Don't let

NOTE

These exercises are not exhaustive and you may add others based on your experience or the advice of a healthcare or fitness professional.

TIPS FROM THE TEAM

3-D Ball Training can help to improve:
- posture
- muscle strength and endurance
- athletic performance
- joint and muscle position sense (kinesthetic awareness)
- ability to dissociate upper and lower extremities
- dynamic balance
- movement efficiency.

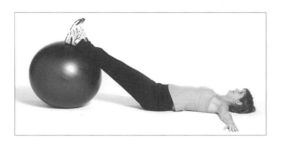

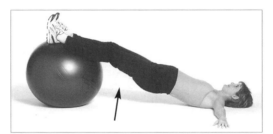

Ball bridges.

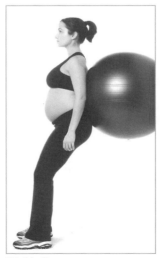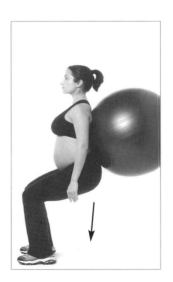

Wall ball squats.

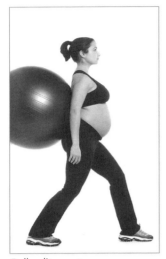 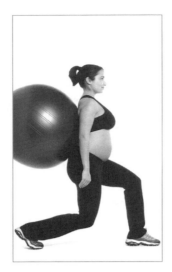

Ball split squats.

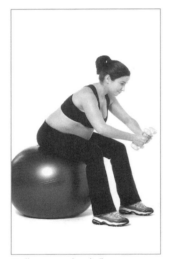 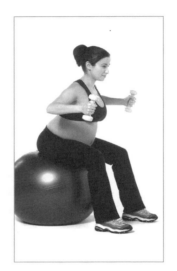

Ball reverse back flys.

 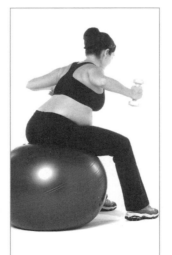

the knees get ahead of the toes. Progress to single leg squats when able.

- Increase leg strength and stability by gradually increasing number of repetitions and depth of the squat.
- Strengthens core, front thigh and buttocks.

Ball Split Squats (ball at back)

- Stand with your feet together, arms at your sides. Fire the core and sustain.
- Step forward until you are in a split position, keeping your back straight and your head up.
- Bend until your front thigh is parallel to the floor, ensuring that at the bottom of the movement your front knee does not pass your toes.
- Your back leg should be almost straight and should not touch the floor. Always exhale on exertion.
- This exercise stretches the hip flexors and improves balance at the same time.
- Hand weights can be added to increase resistance.
- Strengthens core, front thigh and buttocks.

Ball Reverse Back Flys

- Sit on the ball, feet shoulder-width apart.
- Fire the core and sustain.
- Bend forward until abdomen rests on knees.
- Flex elbows to 90 degrees and raise up, squeezing shoulder blades together.
- Add small hand weights as you become stronger.
- Strengthens mid back and shoulders.

Diagonal Hip Flexion (ball at back)

- Place an exercise ball at your mid back against the wall.
- Start in a split squat position with one leg back, and fire the core and sustain.
- Flex the hip so your knee comes up and across at waist height.
- Lower slowly keeping the core fired.
- Strengthens core, front thigh and buttocks.

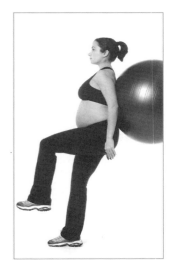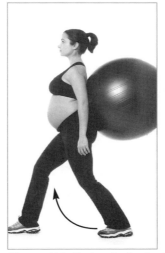

Diagonal hip flexion (ball at back).

Diagonal Hip Flexion (pull ball down in front)

- Hold an exercise ball against the wall.
- Fire the core and sustain.
- Squeeze the ball gently and pull down as you flex hip up.
- Lower slowly, keeping the core fired.
- Strengthens core, front thigh and buttocks.

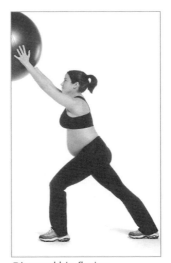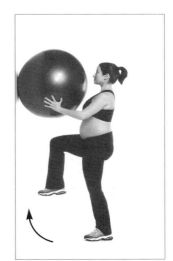

Diagonal hip flexion.

Bicep Curls sitting on the ball

- Sitting on the ball with feet flat on the floor, find your balance point.
- Fire the core and sustain for stability and bend elbow to raise stretch cord or dumbbell up toward shoulder.
- The exercise ball can be used with a number of upper body exercises to add a balance component.
- Strengthens core and arms.

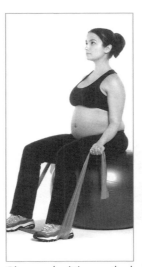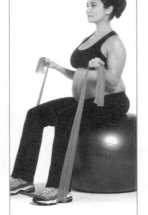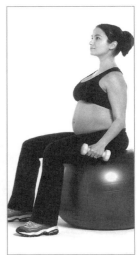

Bicep curls sitting on the ball.

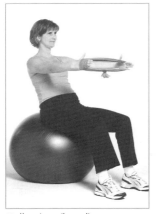 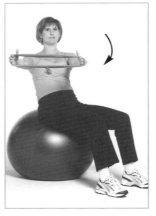 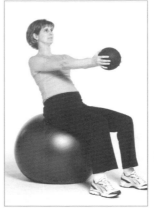 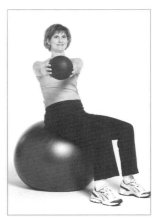

Ball twists (band).   Ball twists (ball).

Ball Twists

- Sit on an exercise ball with your knees bent and feet flat on the floor.
- Fire the core and sustain and lean back, up to 30 degrees.

- Holding a small ball, light weight or stretch cord with straight arms out in front of you, slowly rotate your torso from side to side.

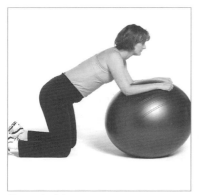 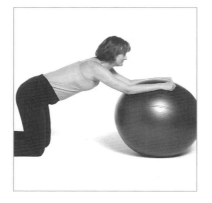 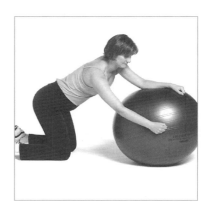

Prayer holds.

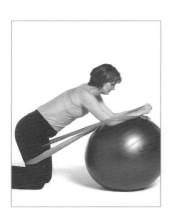 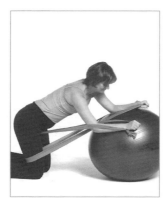

Prayer Holds

- Kneel on the floor with elbows and fore-arms on the ball.
- Fire the core and sustain, and hold for 10 seconds.
- Don't let your back arch. Stop if fatigue sets in.
- By adding stretch cords or rolling the ball to the side you can give your core a more intensive workout.
- Do 2–3 sets of 5–10 repetitions.
- Strengthens core and arms.

Ball Sit Ups-Downs

- Sit on the ball, slightly ahead of center, with your knees bent and feet flat on the floor.
- Cross your arms on your chest, then fire the core and sustain.
- Slowly lean back to 30–40 degrees, letting the ball roll to support your lower back.
- Strengthens core muscles as they lengthen.

Sample Exercise Ball Workouts
Trimester 1
Warm-up

- 15 minutes on an exercise bike or walking on a treadmill.
- Rate of Perceived Exertion: 3–5, or use the talk test.
- Do Dynamic Warm-up exercises (see chapter 5).

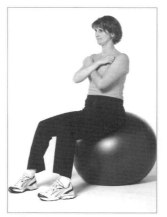
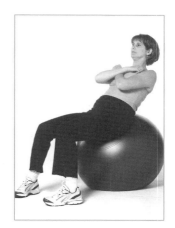

Ball sit downs.

> **NOTE**
>
> *These exercises are not exhaustive and you may add others based on your experience or the advice of a healthcare or fitness professional.*

General Exercise Routine

Choose 4–6 exercises, and change them regularly. Do 1–2 sets of 10–15 repetitions.

- Ball Sitting Dead Bugs
- Wall Ball Squats
- Ball Split Squats (ball at back)
- Diagonal Hip Flexion (ball at back)
- Diagonal Hip Flexion (pull ball down in front)
- Ball Bridges
- Ball Twists
- Ball Sit Ups-Downs (works abdominals as they lengthen)
- Prayer Holds

Upper Body Exercises

Do 1–2 sets of 10–15 repetitions. Any of these exercises can be done sitting on or leaning against the ball to add a balance component. Choose 1–2 exercises for all other muscle groups, and change them regularly.

Back

- Bent Over One-Arm Rows
- Seated Row
- Lat Pulldowns (wide grip) overhand
- Ball Reverse Back Flys

Chest

- Incline Bench Press
- Flat Bench Press (not shown)
- Incline Flys
- Push-ups (with bent knees) (not shown)
- Ball Incline Press (not shown)

Shoulders/Arms

- Lateral Raises, seated
- Front Shoulder Raises, seated
- Bicep Dumbbell Curls

Core (Trunk) and Pelvic Floor Stability

Choose 2–4 exercises, and change them regularly. Add some of your favorite exercises that strengthen the core as well as other muscles.

- Five on the Floor, including Tighten (Fire the Core and Sustain) with Leg Slide, Leg Fall Out (abduction), March and Dying Bug
- 4-Point Kneeling Pony Back to Neutral (suck in your tummy and flatten your back)
- Supine Bridging (stomach up)
- Supine Bridging (with stretch cord abduction)
- Clamshell
- Circus Ponies (alternating arm and leg raises; use ball or on all fours)

Choose 2 exercises
- Kegel exercises including Hold-ems, Speed-ems, Squeeze-ems and Elevate-ems
- Belly Button Breaths (in through nose, out through mouth HA HA HA)
- Baby Hugs (big, bigger, biggest)

To effectively fire the core and sustain you must follow these principles:
- Ensure that the initial contraction is isolated (no other muscles substituting).
- The contraction should begin slowly with control.
- Low effort is all that is required.
- Breathe normally.

Cooldown and Stretching

- Evaluate how you feel. Have a drink of water.
- Concentrate on stretching the pectorals, hamstrings, low back and hip flexors.

Trimesters 2 & 3

Warm-up

- 15 minutes on an exercise bike or walking on a treadmill.
- Rate of Perceived Exertion: 3–5, or use the talk test.
- Do Dynamic Warm-up exercises (see chapter 5).

General Exercise Routine

Choose 4–6 exercises, and change them regularly. Do 1–2 sets of 10–15 repetitions.
- Ball Sitting Dead Bugs
- Wall Ball Squats
- Ball Split Squats (ball at back)
- Diagonal Hip Flexion (ball at back)
- Diagonal Hip Flexion (pull ball down in front)
- Ball Twists
- Ball Sit Ups-Downs (works abdominals as they lengthen)
- Prayer Holds

Upper Body

Do 1–2 sets of 10–15 repetitions. Any of the exercises can be done sitting on or leaning against the ball to add a balance component. Choose 1–2 exercises for all other muscle groups, and change them regularly.

Back
- Bent Over One-Arm Rows
- Seated Row
- Lat Pulldowns (wide grip) overhand

Chest
- Incline Bench Press
- Flat Bench Press (not shown)
- Incline Flys
- Ball Incline Press

Shoulders/Arms
- Lateral Raises, seated
- Front Shoulder Raises, seated
- Bicep Dumbbell Curls

Core (Trunk) and Pelvic Floor Stability

Choose 2–4 exercises, and change them regularly. Add some of your favorite exercises that strengthen the core as well as other muscles.
- Five on the Floor, including Tighten (Fire the Core and Sustain) with Leg Slide, Leg Fall Out (abduction), March and Dying Bug
- Pony Back to Neutral (suck in your tummy and round your back)
- Supine Bridging (stomach up)
- Supine Bridging (with stretch cord abduction)
- Clamshell
- Circus Ponies (alternating arm and leg raises; use ball or on all fours)

Choose 2 exercises
- Kegel exercises including Hold-ems, Speed-ems, Squeeze-ems and Elevate-ems
- Belly Button Breaths (in through nose, out through mouth HA HA HA)
- Baby Hugs (big, bigger, biggest)

To effectively fire the core and sustain you must follow these principles:
- Ensure that the initial contraction is isolated (no other muscles substituting).
- The contraction should begin slowly with control.
- Low effort is all that is required.
- Breathe normally.

Cooldown and Stretching
- Evaluate how you feel. Have a drink of water.
- Concentrate on stretching the pectorals, hamstrings, low back and hip flexors.

9

Relaxation Techniques

By Joanne Timlick, R.N., B.S.N.

Relaxation Exercises
Why should I practice them during pregnancy?

You're about to embark on one of the most exciting periods of your life: pregnancy and birth. It's a time of growth and development that provides you with an opportunity to evaluate your lifestyle and possibly make some changes that may have lifelong health benefits. Many variables influence how you will respond to this time. The ability to incorporate comfort and relaxation techniques into your lifestyle can be a source of relief. As well, active interest from family and friends during pregnancy and labor indicates to a pregnant woman that she is supported. Words, a glance or a touch help to reduce fears and tensions while at the same time empowering you and increasing your confidence.

There are many benefits to be obtained by early and repeated incorporation of comfort and relaxation techniques during your pregnancy. Adaptation of these skills to best suit your needs and preferences is highly recommended. Learning and practicing relaxation techniques can help you to:

- Manage stress.
- Soothe (decrease) tension.
- Conserve energy.
- Cope with some of the discomforts of pregnancy.
- Build your self-confidence.
- Draw on your inner resources during one of the most stressful periods of all—labor and birth.

There are various techniques to try. Some can work in conjunction with others, but total relaxation is the leading concept of comfort during pregnancy and birth; it is the ability to use conditioning, concentration and discipline to recognize and reduce unnecessary muscle tension, while at the same time calming your mind. The more relaxed you are the more endorphins (pleasure hormones) you'll produce, thus supplying yourself with more stamina and endurance for your pregnancy and birth. Your brain is the most powerful relaxation tool of all, so empower yourself to practice and change your response to stress. Studies have proven that women who incorporate relaxation and comfort techniques into their pregnancies and births have better outcomes, so take advantage of these easy and inexpensive skills.

Relaxation techniques to consider:
- Breath awareness.
- Positioning.

Joanne has worked as a labor and delivery room nurse for 27 years. She developed and initiated a childbirth education series for the hospital in which she is employed. She continues to teach in this series and privately to expectant clients.

• Massage therapy.
• Water therapy.

Other methods are effective as well; the main concern is to adapt skills that will best suit your needs and preferences.

Prior to practicing any relaxation techniques:
• Create a peaceful, soothing environment.
• Play some quiet, soothing music.
• Dim the lights and limit distractions.
• Wear loose non-restrictive clothing.
• Empty your bladder.
• Assume a comfortable position (sidelying or sitting up with pillows).
• Now close your eyes.

Breathing and Relaxation Exercise

Take a deep breath in through your nose
Slowly blow the air out through your mouth
Concentrate on your breathing, it's not hurried

Breathe in
Allow the tension to escape from your body as you breathe out
Your muscles are soft and supple
Your breathing has slowed down
Your face is relaxed
Breathing in slowly and blowing the air out gradually

Your eyes are closed
You're feeling sleepy
Your breathing is rhythmic
Your neck and shoulders are relaxed
Your arms are heavy, weightless

Your lungs are slowly being inflated and deflated

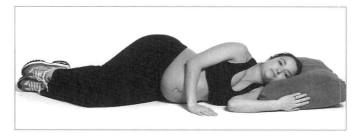

This warm feeling continues down around your abdomen
It embraces your baby, a gentle hug
Breathing slowly in and out
All the tension is totally released from your body

Your pelvic floor muscles are relaxed
Soft and supple
During birth your baby will exit with little resistance
Your legs are heavy and light
A warm, tingling sensation has spread to your feet and toes
You're breathing very slowly

The last bits of tension are being released from your body
Enjoy this feeling of total relaxation
You're drifting…floating…free of discomfort
Your muscles are soft and relaxed
Allow yourself to stay in this state of complete relaxation
Breathing in and out
You have obtained a peaceful and deep state of relaxation

Whenever you feel that it's appropriate take one more deep breath
Start to move your limbs…slowly open your eyes…stretch…yawn
You're feeling empowered, strong and full of energy.

Relaxation and Breathing Tips

- Make this a part of your daily ritual.
- Purchase or create a tape of your own.
- Encourage your partners/coaches to recite this exercise to you.
- Practice your own mental version.
- Feedback and emotional support is encouraged by partners/coaches.
- Practice sessions develop your teamwork and enhance your partner's/coach's tactile and visual acuity of tension and relaxation.

Breath Awareness

The simplified breathing used in the previous exercise is easy to understand and duplicate during your labor. Your breathing should be slow and even so that you avoid hyperventilating, tensing up and feeling out of control. Using this relaxation technique during periods of stress will allow you to get in touch with your body and mind; the two are correlated, so if your body is relaxed you will experience a general sense of well-being. Two opportunities to practice breath awareness are when you are experiencing backache or Braxton-Hicks contractions (false labor pains). Another favorable idea is to practice in different body positions since you will be taking advantage of these when giving birth. Breath awareness is a skill that will help you during your pregnancy, labor and in future stressful situations.

Tips for Practicing Breath Awareness

- Allow your hands to rest lightly on your abdomen.
- Take in a slow, deep, easy breath through your nose.
- As you blow the air out through your mouth feel your abdomen gently press against your hands.
- Continue to breathe in and out slowly.
- Repeat this easy, gentle breathing until you feel that it's appropriate to stop.

Positioning

Practicing and becoming comfortable with different body positions during pregnancy has a number of benefits:

- Different muscle groups are challenged while requiring relaxation in others.
- It may increase comfort while dealing with the discomforts of pregnancy and labor (i.e., backache).
- Practice affords you an opportunity to identify and develop several positions that best reflect your own preferences.
- It widens the diameter of your pelvis, thus aiding in rotating the baby from a posterior position.
- It allows the perineal muscles to relax.
- Other comfort techniques can be used in conjunction with various positions (i.e., counterpressure and massage).
- It can aid in relaxation, rest and sleep.

Three positions to become familiar with:

Hands and Knees: Position yourself on all fours, with pillows underneath your knees and hands to support your body weight. Remain in this position as long as you are comfortable.

Squatting: Hold onto something secure (i.e., a door handle or door frame) and lower yourself into a squat. When practicing with your partner/coach have him/her sit in a chair, and then lower yourself into a squatting position while leaning on him/her for support. If you are considering this position for birth, it is beneficial to practice during pregnancy so that you can maintain this position at various times during your labor.

Sidelying: Lie down, preferably on your left side, with pillows to support your body weight. Bend your legs and arms slightly.

Explore and practice these positions and others but concentrate on those that work best for you.

Massage

The act of contact by your partner/coach with warm, gentle or firm pressure is a soothing, inexpensive and simple tool to use. It is a proven aid for the relief of mind and body tension. Keep in mind, however, that the type of massage you practiced during pregnancy may irritate you during labor, so use whichever technique is comforting at the time.

Tips for Massage

- Assume a comfortable position.
- Use light or firm pressure.
- Be aware of the types of massage strokes that you find comforting and relaxing.
- Use lotions, warmed oil or cornstarch.
- Massage directly against the skin or through light clothing.
- Practice enhances your partner's/coach's tactile and visual acuity of tension and relaxation.

There are a number of different types of massage strokes. Two that you might want to consider are:

- Stroking: Begin the massage with soft, rhythmic strokes over a specific muscle or body part. Start with the tips of your fingers, and then progress to using your hands. Use firm or light pressure in a circular motion. Stroke in one direction.
- Counterpressure: Apply light, firm or direct pressure over the lumbosacral area to relieve backache. During pregnancy, backache is usually due to poor posture or relaxed lower back and pelvic ligaments. During labor, it's usually due to the position that the baby is in or its descent farther into your pelvis. Partners/coaches should stabilize their position during the application by resting their free hand on your hipbone.

Tips for Counterpressure

- Use a variety of aids such as a tennis ball, small paint roller, rolling pin, warmed beanbag or hot water bottle.
- Use a rolling motion during the application of some of the aids.

Water Therapy, Aromatherapy and Music

There is nothing like a long, warm bath to help relieve an aching back! Water has a number of pain-relieving properties:

- It promotes overall relaxation.
- It relieves pressure on aching joints and soft tissues.
- It stimulates touch-sensitive receptors in your skin, producing euphoric feelings similar to those you experience during a massage.
- It promotes relaxation of the pelvic muscles.
- It diminishes the pain associated with contractions.

- It promotes reduced use of analgesics during labor.
- Different body positions can be used in conjunction with water therapy.

Tips for Water Therapy

Darken the room and listen to some of your favorite music. It is not wise to use water therapy if you have leaking or ruptured membranes, so check with your healthcare provider as many prefer that you have a shower rather than a bath. Saunas, hot tubs and hot baths should be avoided due to the risk of overheating.

Music

- Personalize the experience.
- Choose soothing pieces.
- Complement other relaxation techniques with this comfort measure.

Aromatherapy

Consider the guidance of a qualified aromatherapist since certain oils are not recommended during pregnancy and birth.

Yoga and Pilates

Many moms-to-be are already practicing yoga and Pilates. With some minor modifications they are a great way to help prepare your body for childbirth, as Pilates in particular is a good functional workout for the core. Yoga can be a mild form of exercise that nearly every woman can do, with a physician's permission.

Practicing Safe Yoga and Pilates

- Don't push yourself beyond your ability.
- Avoid back extension or twisting movements.
- Avoid poses on the stomach.
- Avoid lying on your back for longer than 30 seconds after the first trimester.
- Avoid exercising in hot environments or in classes where there is no ventilation (sweat yoga is out).
- Drink lots of water.
- Do yoga or Pilates on alternate days; on the other days do some aerobic activity.

Above all, enjoy this time. It truly is a miracle, a birth not only of knowledge but of a life.

Postpartum Guidelines

10

Pre-conception, pregnancy and the postpartum period are very good times to adopt or maintain healthy lifestyle and exercise habits. Combining physical activity with healthy eating promotes a positive approach to life and enhances body image. In addition, by making positive lifestyle choices you are setting a good example for your children and your family.

In general, we talk of the postpartum period lasting for six weeks after birth; many prenatal professionals consider it to last a whole year following delivery. Many of the physiological changes in your body are present until at least six weeks postpartum—for example, some joints will remain hypermobile—so you are advised to continue with your exercise program as if you were still pregnant. By six weeks after delivery you may gradually resume the normal exercise routine that you were doing prior to becoming pregnant. However, your first priority should be caring for your newborn and yourself. As the inevitable sleep deprivation sets in, you are unlikely to have the energy to begin an aggressive exercise program during the first few weeks of your baby's life. As caloric demands increase dramatically in the early postpartum period, be sure to increase your food and water intake. Exercise in addition to the demands of breastfeeding can easily outstrip your food reserves.

In 1994 Dr. James Clapp published the following monitoring guidelines for postpartum women to assist in their return to an exercise program.

1. The woman should exercise three or more times per week.
2. The exercise should feel good and enhance feelings of well-being.
3. There should be no associated pain or heavy bleeding (heavy bleeding is defined as a pad every half hour or bright red bleeding that persists for several hours. If this occurs the woman should cease exercise for at least 48 hours).
4. Fluid intake should be high.
5. Adequate rest is a must.
6. Infant weight gain should be normal.
7. Heavy urine leakage or pelvic pressure during exercise should be assessed.
8. Adequate breast support is vital.

Simple Hints for the Postpartum Period

Improving Your Circulation

You may still have swelling in your extremities (legs and arms) after pregnancy. The following exercises help to promote improved circulation and decrease swelling. (Try doing several sets of 20 repetitions of each exercise every hour.)

• Wrist circles

- Finger squeezes
- Ankle range of motion exercises (draw circles and the alphabet)
- Foot pumps and toe scrunches.

Care of the Perineum

The area between the vagina and anus is made up of muscles and other soft tissue. It may be swollen and painful, or may even have been torn or cut if you had an episiotomy. Doing the following exercises will help minimize the discomfort.

- Pelvic floor exercises (Kegels): Do these 5 times per hour to help improve the healing process and send blood to the area. Squeeze only as hard as is comfortable. See chapter 3 for other Kegel exercises.
- Kegels (pelvis elevated): Try the same Kegel exercise while on your back with two pillows under your pelvis for support, to improve circulation and decrease swelling. This is a good exercise if you have swelling or bruising, a tear or an episiotomy, or if you suffer from hemorrhoids.

The Pelvic Floor

When you increase abdominal pressure by lifting, coughing or sneezing, fire the core and sustain to help protect the pelvic floor. You can also place your hand on your perineum and push upwards when support is needed, or place a rolled-up towel between your legs and pull it up tightly; this is helpful if you are coughing or sneezing frequently. When you feel ready try doing some of the core exercises in chapter 3, like Five on the Floor and More, to help improve control and prepare you for more advanced exercises.

Sitting Comfortably

Swelling and pain may make it uncomfortable to sit. To relieve pressure, place a pillow 6 inches (15 cm) from the back of the chair. Sit down, placing your buttocks between the back of the chair and the pillow while keeping the buttocks squeezed. Once you are sitting, slowly release the buttock muscles and prop up your feet on a stool.

Proper Posture

Correct posture is as important after delivery as before to prevent back pain, and decrease shoulder tension and headaches.

- Sleeping (sidelying): Place a pillow between your knees.
- Sleeping on your back (supine): Place a pillow under your knees.
- When doing activities of daily living, like cooking or washing, elevate one foot on a low stool and fire the core and sustain.
- When breastfeeding ensure your low back is well supported by placing a rolled-up towel behind your back. Bring your baby up to breast level with a pillow rather than resting the baby on your lap and then hunching over.

Proper Breathing

Breathing may have become difficult during the final weeks of your pregnancy because the diaphragm, your main breathing muscle, could not descend fully into your abdomen, which was blocked by your baby. This prevented you taking a full breath and may have changed your breathing pattern.

Physical therapist Diane Lee, author of *PostPartum Health for Moms*, suggests the following breathing exercises:

Lateral Costal Breathing Supine

- Lie on your back with your hips and knees flexed and head comfortably supported with a small towel if necessary.
- Feel your lower anterior ribcage.
- Take a full breath in and expand the lower ribs laterally without bulging the abdomen.
- Move your hands around the sides of your ribcage and repeat this exercise.
- While breathing, pay attention to the action of your pelvic floor. Which way does it move when you breathe in? Which way does it move when you breathe out? Can you feel it move at all?

Lateral Costal Breathing in Cat Position

- Begin by kneeling on all fours, then sit back on your heels with your arms out in front of you.
- Take a deep breath in and focus on opening up the lower ribs as low as you can.
- On the second breath try to send the breath all the way to the pelvic floor.

Post-Caesarean Section Exercises

Following a caesaran section or a traumatic vaginal birth you will need to delay your return to exercise. You must NOT do any heavy lifting, other than your baby, for 6 weeks. You should also avoid doing any aggressive abdominal exercises during this time. Always practice good posture, doing your pelvic tightening and Kegel exercises often to help speed recovery time. Listen to your body, and stop any activity or exercise that causes pain. Avoid bouncy or jerky sudden movements.

Following caesarean surgery the pain and discomfort you experience may cause shallow breathing, reducing the amount of air entering the base of your lungs. If you have had a general anaesthetic it may also cause increased mucus production in the lungs, decreasing airflow. To check, bend your knees up and give two effective huffs. Perform the exercises above to restore normal breathing. The risk of blood clotting in the legs is also greater following surgery, so ankle pumping exercises are important to increase blood flow.

Postpartum Exercises
How soon can I...?

Before resuming any exercise, check with your doctor. If you were at a high fitness level before and during your pregnancy, you may be able to start exercising sooner than if you were at a low or moderate fitness level. But no matter what your fitness level, remember to start exercising slowly. Try doing your third-trimester workout.

Exercising with Baby

Instead of leaving your baby with someone else while you work out, why not include him or her in your exercise program? Your baby will enjoy this one-on-one time together, and you'll improve your strength and conditioning. Exercising moms should always practice good posture (see chapter 3), and ensure that the pelvic floor (PF) and core is contracted or firing during all exercises (see chapter 3). The number of repetitions and sets you perform should be based on your fitness level; in general, 1 or 2 sets of 10–15 repetitions is a good start. If you're feeling strong you can push the baby in a stroller while you walk/jog, or go for a brisk walk with the baby in a front or back carrier (depending on baby's head control). The following exercises can be done at home with your newborn close by.

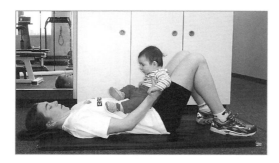

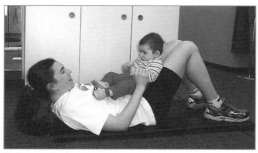

Baby peek-ups.

Always Fire the Core and Sustain

Before each exercise, focus on the following:

- Contract the pelvic floor (Kegel).
- Contract the TA (lower abdominal).
- Remember to breathe.
- Keep knees soft if standing.

Baby Peek-ups

- Lie on your back with knees bent and feet flat on the floor.
- Place baby tummy-down on your abdomen or sit him on your belly, propped up against your thighs.
- Inhale, then exhale as you fire the core and sustain and lift shoulder blades off the floor.
- Hold, then slowly lower. Repeat 10–15 times.
- Strengthens abdominals (lower and upper).

Activity	After vaginal delivery	After a C-section
Do Kegels	From day 1	From day 1
Walk around the block	As soon as you feel comfortable	As soon as you feel comfortable
Do ab exercise	2 weeks, with doctor's OK	6 weeks, with doctor's OK
Do yoga	2 weeks, with doctor's OK	6 weeks, with doctor's OK
Lift weights	2 weeks, with doctor's OK	6 weeks, with doctor's OK
Jog	3–4 weeks	10–12 weeks
Ride a bike	Wait for doctor's approval	Wait for doctor's approval
Kick box	Wait for doctor's approval	Wait for doctor's approval
Do low-impact aerobics	6 weeks	8–12 weeks
Use the stairclimber	6 weeks	8–12 weeks
Run a 5k	6–8 weeks	12–16 weeks
Run a 10k	12–16 weeks	12–16 weeks

Kneeling Cat Backs (not shown)

- Lie baby on his back and kneel over him, on all fours.
- Exhale while rounding your back, pulling belly button to spine, and then return to neutral.
- Hold for 5–10 seconds and repeat 10–15 times.
- Strengthens core.

Kneeling Moving Lunge

- Place baby on his back between your front foot and back knee, then fire the core and sustain.
- Bending on one knee, slide hips and torso forward to stretch the back leg and strengthen the front lunge leg.
- Move slowly and stop when you feel tension. Repeat 10–15 times.
- Strengthens legs and core.

Wide Stance Good Mornings

- Stand with feet wide apart and knees slightly bent.
- Place baby on the floor in front of you.
- Bend forward to stretch low back and back of legs, then fire the core and sustain.
- Repeat 10–15 times.
- Strengthens legs, back and core.

NOTE

These exercises are not exhaustive and you may add others based on your experience or on the advice of your healthcare or fitness professional.

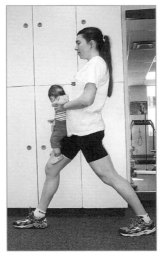
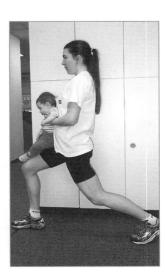

Kneeling moving lunge.

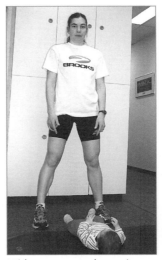
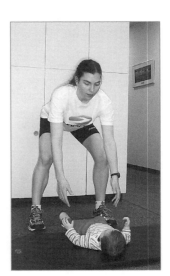

Wide stance good mornings.

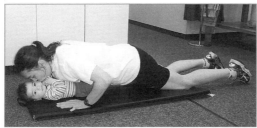

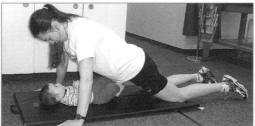

Baby push-ups.

Baby Push-ups

- Kneel in front of your baby and assume the knee push-up position.
- Fire the core and sustain and bend down to touch baby with your face, then push back up.
- When you finish the push-up your elbows should form a 90-degree angle.
- Try these with arms placed at narrow, medium and wide widths.
- Strengthens arms, shoulders and chest.

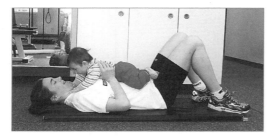

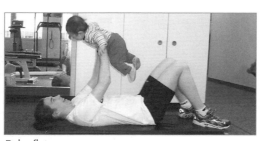

Baby flat press-ups.

Baby Flat Press-ups

- Lie flat on your back holding your baby. Fire the core and sustain.
- Press baby up toward ceiling and lower slowly.
- Repeat 10–15 times.
- Strengthens arms, shoulders and chest.

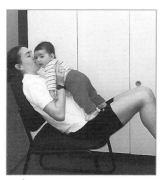
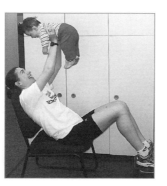

Incline press-ups.

Incline Press-ups

- Lie in an incline position with your back supported by a pillow or ball or sit in a chair, then fire the core and sustain.
- Press baby up toward ceiling, then lower back to your chest and give her a kiss.
- Repeat 10–15 times.
- Strengthens arms, shoulders and chest.

Mini Squats

- You may carry your baby for resistance, or place baby on the floor below you.
- Making sure that knees track over toes, fire the core and sustain, then lower slowly and contract your gluteals as you slowly stand up.
- Repeat 10–15 times.
- Strengthens legs, buttocks and abdominals.

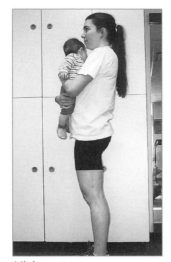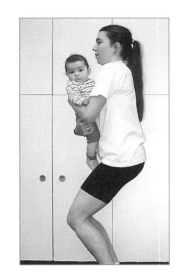

Mini squats.

Sumo Squats

- You may carry your baby for resistance, or place baby on the floor below you.
- Making sure that knees track over toes, fire the core and sustain, then lower slowly and contract your gluteals as you slowly stand up.
- Repeat 10–15 times.
- Strengthens leg muscles, back and abdominals.

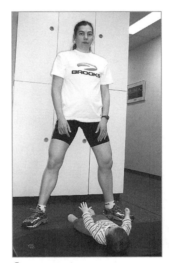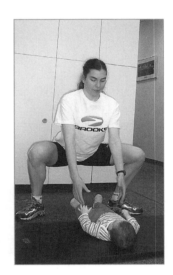

Sumo squats.

Hip Bridges (baby on hips)

- Lie on your back with knees bent and feet hip-width apart.
- Place baby face up on your pelvis.
- Fire the core and sustain, and exhale as you lift hips up to straight.
- Uncurl your spine to the floor.
- Do with feet and knees both narrow and hip-width apart.
- Hold for 5 seconds and repeat 10–15 times.
- Strengthens back, buttocks and pelvic floor muscles.

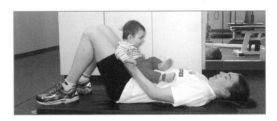

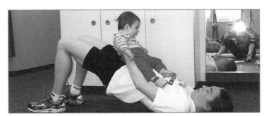

Hip bridges.

Hip Bridges (with stretch cord abduction) (shown on page 23)

- On a mat, lie on your back with feet on the floor and knees bent to 90 degrees. Knees should be aligned directly over the toes and about hip-width apart.
- Keep the head and arms relaxed.
- Place a stretch cord around your knees.

- Fire the core and sustain, pushing knees apart against the stretch cord and lifting hips as above.
- Weight should be on the upper back, not the neck.
- Hold for 4 seconds and do 2–3 sets of 10–15 repetitions.
- Strengthens core and hips.

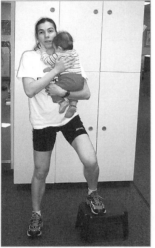
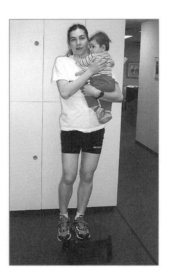

Step-ups (side).

Step-ups (front or side)

- Stand facing a stool, then fire the core and sustain and pull shoulders back.
- Hold your baby for resistance, or hold a dumbbell in each hand.
- Exhale as you step up onto a stool, ensuring that the stool you are stepping onto is not placing your knee beyond 90 degrees.
- Strengthens legs, buttocks and abdominals.

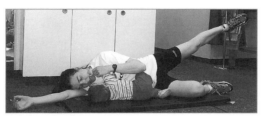
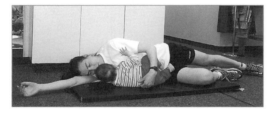

Sidelying leg lifts.

Sidelying Leg Lifts

- Lie on right side with your right hand supporting head. Place left hand on floor in front of your tummy, cradling your baby.
- Fire the core and sustain.
- Keeping your hips forward and toes to the ceiling, raise your leg 8–10 inches and return to starting position.
- Repeat on the opposite side.
- Strengthens lateral hips, back, buttocks and pelvic floor muscles.

Seated Good Mornings

- Sit on the edge of a chair or bench holding baby close to your chest.
- Place feet and knees more than shoulder-width apart, and fire the core and sustain.
- Lean forward from the waist as you exhale and lower your torso.
- Return to upright and repeat 10–15 times.
- Strengthens upper and lower back.

Stroller or Backpack Walking Lunges (not shown)

- While carrying baby in the backpack or pushing her in the stroller, fire the core and sustain, then step forward and lunge.
- Knees should bend no farther than 90 degrees and should track in line with the toes.
- Try sets of 10–15 repetitions.
- Strengthens legs, back and abdominals.

Carriers

A wide range of infant carriers is now available so western parents can enjoy the advantages that other cultures have had for centuries. Transporting the baby in a carrier leaves your hands free, and the baby feels the reassurance of your body motion. The infant is upright which aids digestion, and babies carried this way apparently cry less as they may feel safer.

You may find back carriers more comfortable, but for the first few months you must carry your baby in a front carrier until he or she gains strong head control. Avoid carrying your infant on one hip for any length of time, as this causes your spine to twist and can lead to mal-alignment compensations. As well, carrying your baby on one shoulder causes imbalance and in-

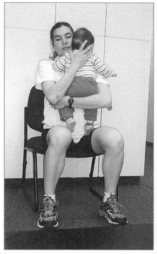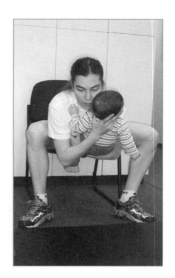

Seated good mornings.

creases the lumbar curve (hollow) in your lower back which stresses the joints.

For front carriers/slings: Your child should be comfortable, well supported and able to breathe freely. Position the baby in the middle of your body and close to your center of gravity.

For back carriers: Loosen the straps so that the baby sits around your waist, taking his or her weight near your center of gravity. Often parents place the back pack too high, challenging balance and increasing the load on their joints. It's best to have the baby ride in the center of your back, as you would ride a horse.

45-Minute Fitness

Getting back into shape will improve your quality of life and make your activities of daily living and sports more enjoyable. But you may be having trouble fitting a lengthy workout into your daily schedule while caring for a newborn. Lack of time is a common problem for many people, especially new moms, so here's a quick 45-minute workout guaranteed to boost your fitness.

You can do this workout anywhere, and all you need is running gear and 45 minutes of free time. Vary the route you run, and use forest trails or waterside paths to prevent wear and tear on your joints and boost your psyche. Taking a friend will encourage you to follow through regularly. When winter weather arrives a treadmill or stationary bike can substitute for the running portion.

Begin with a *slow warm-up jog* for 5 minutes that includes some *dynamic mobility exercises* such as arm circles, leg swings, crossover runs, backward running, side shuffle steps and skipping. These exercises improve agility and coordination at the same time as warming up the muscles of the shoulder girdle, hips and pelvis.

Do some *continuous running* until you reach the 18-minute mark, keeping your heart rate at between 65–75% of maximum [maximum heart rate = 220 – your age] or at an RPE (rate of perceived exertion) of 6–7 out of 10. This ensures that you get a good aerobic benefit.

On we go!

Next do alternating sets of *mini squats* and *stride lunges*.

Mini squats are very functional and provide both concentric (shortening) and eccentric (lengthening) muscle contractions. They

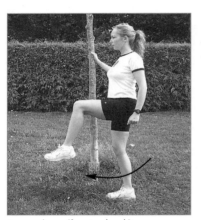
Leg swings (front – back)

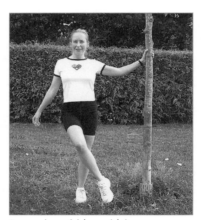
Leg swings (side – side)

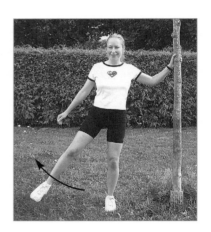

Crossover runs, high knees, high heels and skips will not only loosen your hips, but keep you quick on your feet.

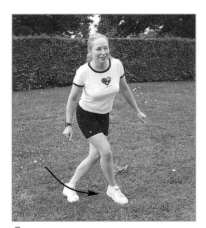
Crossovers.

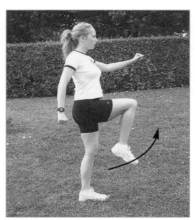
High knees.

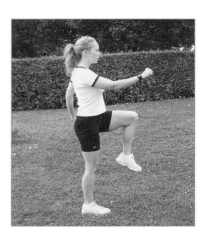

stimulate the medial quadriceps to work, and strengthening these helps maintain proper knee alignment and may decrease knee pain that is associated with muscular imbalances.

Alternate mini squats with sets of *stride lunges*. Stride lunges improve flexibility in the hip flexors and extensors, improve balance and coordination in the hip, knee and ankle, and increase strength in the hips and legs. Keeping your back straight and head up, take your rear knee down toward the ground.

Start slowly with 2–3 sets of 10–20 repetitions, going only to a 30–45 degree knee angle. Over the period of a month, gradually increase until you can do sets of 20–30 repetitions.

Mini squats and stride lunges also help decrease your risk of injury by dynamically correcting potential imbalances in your pelvis, hips and legs. Not a bad pay-off for a few minutes' work!

Continue *jogging* until you reach the 35–40 minute mark, then start walking to cool down.

Cooling Down

While cooling down, add a little more *general body strength* to the workout by alternating the following exercises. Move from one exercise to the next without resting to continue the aerobic benefits.

Sit Downs

Work your core functionally by starting in a sit up position and doing a reverse crunch or sit down.

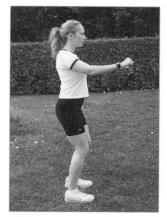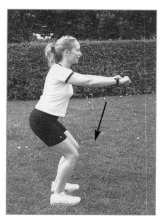

Mini squats — Keep knees aligned over your toes. Try to maintain a high arch as you go down. Start slowly to gain control of the knee and after several sessions gradually progress to a faster drop and then increase from double to single leg.

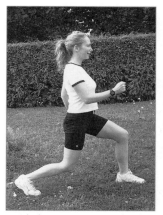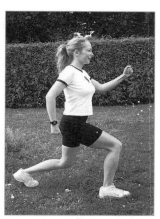

Stride lunges — Start slowly and easily to ensure no muscle strains.

NOTE

If you suffer from groin pain avoid stride lunges until cleared by your caregiver.

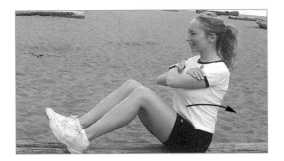

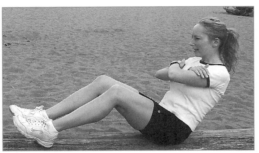

Sit downs.

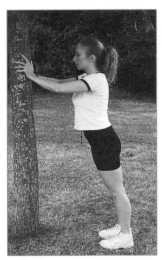

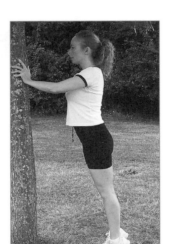

Calf raises.

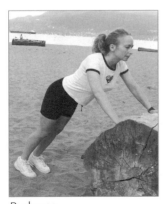

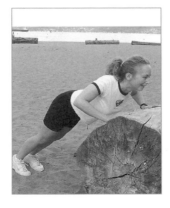

Push-ups.

Calf Raises

Work all lower leg muscles. Raise up slowly, hold for 2 seconds, and lower slowly. Try for 2 × 10–20.

Push-ups

Improve the strength of the chest muscles and shoulder stabilizers. Do one set of push-ups in each of three different hand positions: hands narrow (thumbs touching), shoulder-width, and wide. When starting out try doing them in a kneeling position or against a table to decrease the resistance.

Hip Bridges

Lying on your back with knees bent to 90 degrees, bridge hips up in the air and hold for 4 seconds. Do 2–3 sets of 10–15 repetitions.

Now the 45 minutes are up and your workout is finished. Head for the showers and still have time for a quick lunch or to make

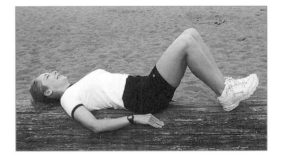

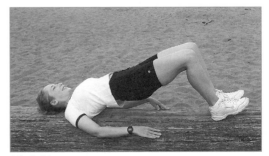

Hip bridges.

dinner. Add some variety by changing the agility exercises you do at the beginning, changing the cardio (aerobic) component from cycle to stairclimber or elliptical trainer, or by changing the general body exercises.

Cross-Training

When organizing your training schedule, include a variety of methods for training different energy systems and activating different muscle groups. Cross-training also presents the opportunity for new challenges to the musculo-skeletal and cardio-respiratory systems. An added benefit is injury prevention: by using cross-training methods that are non-weight bearing you reduce the wear and tear on your joints and muscles. Be sure to vary your route or training environment, and you may also find that changing training partners can stimulate fresh training ideas. Allow yourself occasional unstructured training or active rest. Play a game like soccer or tennis with little regard for intensity, and use it as an easy stamina workout in your plan.

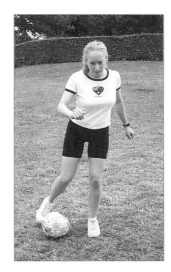

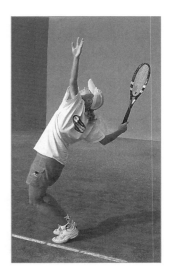

NOTE *On rainy days consider using an indoor piece of aerobic equipment such as a stationary cycle, stairclimber or rowing machine. You will stay warmer and get a better workout with no coasting and no lights.*

Quick Calorie Burners

Having trouble squeezing in your workouts between a hectic work and family schedule? Following are five quick workouts to help boost your fitness and burn a few calories.

Treadmill Walking: A 10-minute walk at a 15 minute per mile pace with a 10% incline burns approximately 70 calories. Using a treadmill on the incline maximizes your calorie expenditure as well as providing less stress on the joints. The uphill walking burns about 70% more calories than level walking. Start easy and gradually in-

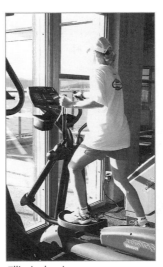

Elliptical trainer.

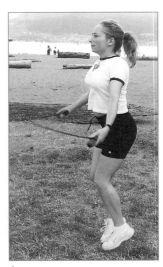

Jump rope.

crease the speed and the grade. If you have to hang on to the rails the treadmill is going too fast and you're burning fewer calories.

Elliptical Trainer or Cross-Country Ski Machine: Ten minutes at a moderate level burns approximately 90 calories. As your technique on this machine improves you will burn more calories from your increased range of motion. To help improve your glide

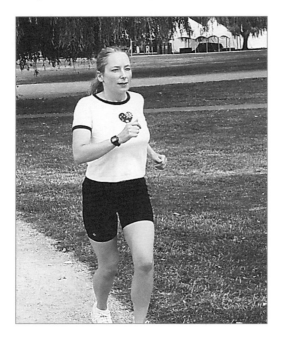

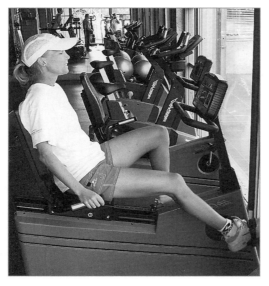

motion lift your heel at the end of the stride. Alternate your routine between short quick steps and long smooth glides to vary the intensity.

Rowing: Ten minutes using a setting that is somewhat hard burns approximately 70 calories. Initiate the move from your legs and buttocks, not your back and arms, and maintain a smooth continuous stroke with no stopping or hesitation.

Jump Rope: Doing ten consecutive minutes of rope skipping is more strenuous than it looks. Instead start with interval jumping, alternating 20–30 jumps with 20–30 steps of in-place marching. As your coordination and stamina improve gradually increase the rope jumping and decrease the marching. Burns approximately 90 calories.

Stationary Bike: Keep your pedal speed high (80–90 RPMs) for the full 10 minutes but alternate the resistance setting to increase the intensity of the workout. Try a ladder climb of 30, 45, 60, 60, 45, 30 seconds of hard pedaling, following each one with an equal amount of time just spinning at a high RPM. Burns approximately 80 calories.

Speed Play (Fartlek)

To add variety to your program, try fartlek training. Fartlek training originated in Scandinavia, and translated simply means "speed play." By varying the route and using hilly terrain, you perform sections of the workout at a higher aerobic power and/or anaerobic intensity. This makes your stamina more sport specific. As well, you can add a speed and agility component by using natural obstacles. A good forest run of this type can be a great rejuvenator of the spirit while giving you a good workout. This can also be done with cycling or swimming by either changing gears or strokes. Speed hiking or in-line skating are also excellent ways to improve general aerobic and anaerobic stamina and build some strength endurance at the same time.

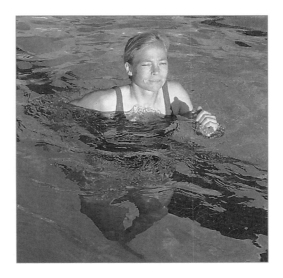

Sample Fartlek Programs

Fartlek Running

- Jog 10 minuntes to warm up, then do 4–5 minutes of light calisthenics and stretches.
- Run 2 × 2 minutes at a fast pace 70%, walking 2 minutes after each.
- Do 3 × 200m acceleration sprints (jog 50m, stride 50m, sprint 50m, walk 50m). Sprint 3 × 100m at 80%, jogging 100m between each.
- Walk 2–3 minutes. Run slow × 2 minutes.
- Run 2 × 400m at 80%, jogging slowly for 400m between each.
- Walk 2–3 minutes.
- Run slow 7–8 minutes for a cooldown.

In-Line Skating

Keep your fitness "in line" with a blade workout. Warm up with 15 minutes steady skating, then do some crossovers, agility and balance work. Once you are warm do a hard 8 × 4 program: skate hard for 8 strides then make 4 medium radius turns (generating speed). Repeat 8 times for 1 set. If your fitness allows try to do 4–8 sets.

Cycling Intervals

Here is a riding workout guaranteed to quicken the pulse and strengthen the legs. Do 2–4 repeats of repetitions of 30/60/90/

120/90/60/30 seconds keeping your heart rate at 80–85% of maximum (RPE of 7–8), during exercise and decreasing to 120 beats/min. between reps (RPE of 3–4). Rest between sets until heart rate goes below 100 beats/min.

Fartlek Water Running

- Jog easy × 3 minutes.
- Do 5 × 20 seconds full out, slow treading 1 minute between each.
- Ladder run at 80% of maximum heart rate for 30/45/60/75/90/75/60/45/30 seconds (rest interval of 50% work time) (RPE = 7–8).
- Tread slow × 3 minutes.
- Fast runs 2 × 3 reps of 60 seconds (rest interval 30 seconds between reps and 60 seconds between sets).
- Cooldown walk in shallow end × 4 minutes.

Postpartum Tune-up

Worried that you haven't run farther than across the street or for the bus in the last few weeks? Here are several sure-fire workouts to get you back in shape, regardless of your current level of fitness.

To ensure success in your training program, follow these principles:

- **Regular participation.** You should aim for at least 4 to 6 days per week.
- **Overload.** The training load must be high enough to tax the body's systems during a workout, to promote increased efficiency in the transport of oxygen and blood to the working muscles, and to improve strength, endurance and power in the muscles. The duration of the activity must be long enough to produce a training effect, and the intensity of the workouts must increase in a gradual and logical manner.
- **Rest and recovery.** It is important to allow your body's tissues, including the central nervous system, time to recover from the fatigue caused by training.
- **Flexibility.** Remain flexible in the planning of your workouts. Be in control of your fitness, but don't be a slave to it.
- **Keep it fun.** Training should be fun and stimulating. If you're not enjoying yourself, make some changes to your program.

Training Stamina (Energy Systems)

Your body has three different energy systems—anaerobic alactic, lactic and aerobic—that work together to provide energy to the working muscles.

The anaerobic alactic system does not require oxygen. It uses energy stored in the muscle cells for fuel and does not produce lactic acid. It is the primary energy source for activities that last up to 15 seconds of maximum effort—very important for running after a stray toddler!

The anaerobic lactic system also requires no oxygen, but uses carbohydrates for fuel and produces lactic acid. It is the primary energy source for activities lasting from 15 seconds to 2 minutes. If you're getting into shape to play an intense racquet sport like squash or tennis you will want to train this energy system.

The aerobic system requires oxygen, uses fats and carbohydrates for fuel and does not produce lactic acid. It is the primary source of energy for activities lasting more than 2 minutes. It is also a very important base for all other aspects of your fitness regimen.

Stamina Training Smarts (Aerobic and Anaerobic)

Aerobic endurance and power should be developed before anaerobic endurance. A solid base of aerobic endurance facilitates recovery and allows training at higher intensity levels. A good aerobic base will help improve your anaerobic and strength training because it helps promote faster recovery.

Stamina Principles

Maximum aerobic fitness is genetically limited, and even with training most people will not improve more than 30%. Begin gradually, especially after a long layoff period, and increase slowly, adding no more than 10–15% volume (amount) per week to avoid overuse injuries such as tibial stress syndrome, patello-femoral pain or plantar fasciitis.

Use It or Lose It

Aerobic capacity (stamina) is lost rapidly when training is stopped. The gain produced by 3 months of training is lost in 6 weeks without training, so try to work out consistently at least 2 times per week.

Alternate Hard-Easy Sessions

If you're training more than 4 days per week, alternate hard and easy sessions. Your body's tissues and energy supply require adequate time to recover, and the hard days deplete muscle glycogen which takes 48 hours to replenish.

Start Smart with a Walk-Jog

If you are just beginning to run as a form of training or if you are recovering from injury, this program is a safe and effective start.

Warm up with a fast walk or other continuous activity. When you have broken a light sweat do some dynamic warm-up exercises described in chapter 5.

Start with a fast daily walk and work up to 20 minutes of continuous walking.

Once you can walk briskly for 20 minutes you are ready to begin the walk-jog program.

Healthy Weight and Eating Guidelines Postpartum

Understandably, many new moms are anxious to get back to their pre-pregnancy weight as quickly as possible. It is important to note that rates of weight loss after pregnancy are variable. Most women return to within 2 to 4 pounds (1 to 2 kilograms) of their pre-pregnancy weight by one year postpartum, while women who gained weight beyond the recommended range are more likely to take longer to lose the weight. Breastfeeding is recommended as the optimal method of feeding your baby for up to the first year, and you can expect to

lose about 2 to 4 pounds (1 to 2 kilograms) per month while breastfeeding. Although breastfeeding and returning to your regular exercise program will enhance weight loss, you should avoid strict dieting.

There has been no reproducible study demonstrating that exercise has a negative effect on the quality or quantity of breast milk. The most important determinant of your breast milk quality appears to be how much fluid you drink. Even when women participated in a moderately intense exercise program while breastfeeding, there was no change in milk production providing they stayed adequately hydrated.

Just as when you were pregnant, you are the source of nourishment for your baby and will want to make quality food choices while breastfeeding. Your nutritional requirements while breastfeeding are similar to those during pregnancy: you will need up to an extra 450 calories per day and should ensure you are getting enough protein (up to 20 extra grams per day) and calcium (1500 mg per day) while maintaining a good iron and folic acid intake. To minimize the discomfort of gas for your baby, you may want to consider avoiding heavily spiced foods, high-fat or greasy foods and potentially gas-causing vegetables such as cabbage, broccoli and even raw carrots. Caffeine and alcohol pass readily into breast milk. Caffeine may cause irritability and even insomnia in both you and your baby and should be limited; avoid alcohol if possible. Most medications will pass into breast milk, and even a laxative you have taken could contribute to diarrhea in your baby. It is important to check with your doctor and pharmacist if you have any doubts about any medications—

prescription or over-the-counter—that you are taking.

For additional information on nutrition during pregnancy and the first year of your baby's life, contact www.eatingforenergy.com.

Eating Well: Nutritional Guidelines During Pregnancy
Written by Patricia Chuey, M.Sc., RDN
www.eatingforenergy.com

For more information see Patricia Chuey, M.Sc., R.D.N., *The 80–20 Cookbook— Eating for Energy Without Deprivation*
www.eatingforenergy.com

What Should I Eat During Pregnancy?

By Patricia Chuey

It is important to eat a healthy, balanced diet during pregnancy. Although just 100 extra calories per day will do in your first trimester, you will need to consume approximately 300 extra calories per day in order to support your growing baby and your own nutritional needs, including any additional demands from an exercise program. You should ensure that you derive approximately 25–30% of your calories from quality fats, needed to provide the baby with essential fatty acids (found in fish, olive, canola and flax oil) for proper development. Taking a prenatal supplement can help ensure you are meeting your nutrient requirements. Many women think they can simply take two vitamins if they did not eat well that day, but this is not recommended since foods contain many valuable nutrients not found in supplements. As well, the nutrients consumed through food are generally better absorbed than those from supplements. Since individual needs for calories and nutrients vary based on height, weight and level of activity, talk with a registered dietitian if you have concerns about whether or not you are getting enough. This is of extra importance if you are a teenager or an elite athlete training at a high level, you have many food allergies or you follow a strict vegetarian diet.

The average weight gain during pregnancy is 24 to 30 pounds (11 to 14 kilo-grams). Although you may find it difficult to accept the changes in your weight and body shape, be assured that you will later lose the extra weight through healthy eating, breast-feeding and exercise once the baby is born. It is crucial not to diet or restrict your caloric intake in an effort to limit healthy weight gain, as women who do not gain enough weight are at increased risk of delivering a low birthweight baby (weighing less than 5½ pounds or 2500 grams). Low birth weight is associated with developmental problems and other illnesses.

It is not difficult to obtain enough nutrients during pregnancy if you follow the higher end of the ranges in the USDA's Food Pyramid (available online at www.eatright. org/fgp.html) or Canada's Food Guide to Healthy Eating (available online at www. hc-sc.gc.ca). This includes 5 or more servings per day of grain products, 5 or more servings of vegetables and fruits, 3 to 4 servings of milk products and 2 to 3 servings of meat or meat alternatives. In a very general sense, you can consider the size of a tennis ball or a medium orange to represent one serving (roughly half a cup). Choose whole grains more often and a good variety of fruits and vegetables. When snacking, try to include nutrient-dense foods. For example, choose natural peanut butter or cheese with whole grain bread or crackers and some fruit; yogurt; oatmeal date squares instead of cookies; and fruit salads or milk-based puddings instead of a chocolate bar. Work on establishing a routine of regular meals and snacks (see page 143 for examples) and ensuring you are eating enough food in total.

The nutrient requirements that increase the most during pregnancy include zinc, iron (especially in the third trimester), vitamin B6 and folic acid. It is also important to get enough essential fatty acids. A list of good food sources of these nutrients follows.

Important Nutrients During Pregnancy

- Zinc: oysters, meat, yogurt, fortified cereals and whole grains.
- Iron: lean beef, clams, poultry (dark meat), fish, enriched cereals, cream of wheat, whole grains, beans and lentils, tofu and dark green vegetables.
- Vitamin B6: meat, fish, poultry, grains and cereals, green leafy vegetables, bananas, potatoes and soybeans.
- Folic acid: leafy greens, broccoli and other cruciferous vegetables (cabbage family), oranges, orange juice, legumes and lentils, avocados and fortified food products.
- Essential fatty acids: fish and fish oils, walnuts, flaxseed, olive and canola oils.

The only nutrients you don't need to increase are vitamin A (high levels can be toxic), phosphorus and vitamin D.

In a healthy, perfectly balanced diet you would not need additional calcium during pregnancy. However, most women do not get the recommended 1000 to 1500 milligrams each day, so expectant mothers generally have to increase their calcium intake. Calcium is essential for the development of the baby's bones and teeth, so be sure to consume 4 servings of dairy products each day. One serving is equivalent to 1 cup (250 mL) of milk or fortified soy milk, ¾ cup (175 mL) of yogurt or 1½ ounces (50 g) of cheese, each of which supplies about 250 milligrams of calcium. There is also calcium, although in lesser amounts, in broccoli, kale, bok choy, oranges, almonds and canned fish with bones. If you take calcium in supplemental form, ensure it contains vitamin D to optimize absorption of calcium from the blood into the tissues and bone cells.

Foods to Avoid During Pregnancy

During pregnancy it is important to avoid certain foods and substances that can cross the placenta and enter the baby's bloodstream, where they may harm your developing baby. Aim to quit smoking. If you are having a difficult time quitting, decreasing the number of cigarettes smoked does help but complete cessation is best. Minimize your alcohol intake or, preferably, abstain from drinking altogether. Limit your caffeine intake to less than 300 milligrams per day; this is equal to approximately two or fewer cups of coffee. Be sure to consider your tea intake also, as one cup contains about 50 to 100 milligrams of caffeine. Some less common herbal teas have been shown to cause complications so be careful to drink them in moderation. Those to avoid include pennyroyal, devil's claw, rue, Scotch broom, goldenseal and sassafras. Other teas or herbal products may also be harmful so it is best to consume only moderate amounts or forgo them entirely. Sugar substitutes, such as aspartame, have been approved by Health Canada at a safety level of 40 milligrams per kilogram of body weight per day, but it is advisable to minimize your intake of chemical and artificial foods and beverages during pregnancy and lactation.

Always check with your health professional if you have any doubts about any products you wish to use during pregnancy.

Preventing Food Poisoning

It is especially important to prevent food poisoning during pregnancy. When food is not handled properly, harmful bacteria can grow that can make you and your baby sick. Classic signs of food poisoning include nausea, vomiting, diarrhea or flu-like symptoms. To minimize the risk of food poisoning, always wash your hands before eating anything. Take measures to prevent cross-contamination when preparing food, especially when handling raw meat. Ensure meat is properly cooked, and use a meat thermometer to gauge doneness. Store food safely and use clean surfaces and utensils for food preparation.

Listeria monocytogenes is a bacteria that can be found in soft cheeses, unpasteurized dairy products and undercooked meats and seafood. For this reason, it is advisable to avoid soft cheeses like feta, Brie, Camembert or blue-veined cheeses like Roquefort. If you do eat soft cheeses during pregnancy, it is best to cook them until bubbly. You can still enjoy hard cheeses like cheddar and mozzarella. Cream cheese and yogurt (a valuable source of calcium during pregnancy) are also acceptable. Other foods to avoid include raw seafood and raw shellfish (be careful with sushi), pâtés, unpasteurized fruit juices or ciders and raw eggs (ask at restaurants if you suspect raw eggs may

have been used in a smoothie or Caesar salad dressing, and avoid licking the spoon for homemade cookies or cakes that use eggs). As always, be careful with any foods that may have been left out of the fridge for more than one hour, especially during warm weather. Of particular concern are egg-based mayonnaise and salad dressings, whipped cream, meat and dairy products. Cold ready-to-eat meats like uncooked hot dogs, smoked salmon, bologna or other deli meats should either be thoroughly heated or avoided. It is also wise to avoid questionable street vendors or restaurants you have never tried before.

Mercury in Fish

Due to concerns about exposure to high levels of mercury, shark, marlin and swordfish should be avoided while pregnant and while breastfeeding. Tuna should be restricted to a maximum of one can or one fresh steak per week. Other fresh fish, properly cooked, is fine and provides a lean source of quality protein and fat for you and your growing baby.

Minimizing Allergies

Allergies occur when the body's immune system reacts to normally safe substances. Unfortunately, the prevalence of allergies in both children and adults is increasing with the ever-expanding array of allergens, chemicals and toxins in our environment and food supply. If you or your partner has allergies or a strong family history of allergies, your baby may inherit the tendency to develop allergies; however, this depends on both genetic and environmental factors.

Good evidence exists to suggest that a

baby's sensitivity to allergens may actually begin during pregnancy, at as early as 22 weeks' gestation. The more you suffer from allergic reactions during your pregnancy, the greater chance your baby has of developing allergies. To help prevent allergies in your baby, minimize your exposure to the foods or environmental factors that trigger an allergy. Reducing exposure to dust, cigarette smoke and other environmental toxins is good advice, even for pregnant women without a strong history of allergies.

If you have extensive food allergies, meet with your doctor and a dietitian to assist in keeping your diet well-balanced while avoiding any suspect foods. Even without an allergy to nuts, it is prudent to avoid nuts during pregnancy and breastfeeding.

Managing Discomfort

Pregnancy can be a wonderful time but many women suffer from unpleasant symptoms, most often in the first and last weeks. Following are a few suggestions for relief from some common complaints.

Nausea

Eat small, frequent meals. Eat slowly and chew your food well. If possible, avoid mixing hot and cold foods in the same meal. Try to avoid the strong smells associated with cooking food. Room temperature meals are often easiest to handle as they have less odor than hot foods. Do not drink fluids with meals or snacks but rather in between. To settle your stomach, try nibbling on crackers or dry toast before getting out of bed in the morning. Limit fatty or fried foods. Drink fluids like flat ginger ale, clear tea or apple juice. Let fresh air into your home. Consider adding a squeeze of lemon to your water or eating lemon-flavored yogurt at breakfast. When you do feel hungry and are able to eat, think about what would be most appealing to you. Earthy foods like brown rice and mushrooms, crunchy foods like celery and apples, bland foods such as mashed potatoes and specific sweet or salty items such as plain cookies or pretzels may be easiest to keep down. Cool foods without a strong aroma, such as fruit-based popsicles, gelatin desserts and dry cereal, may also be well tolerated.

Acid Reflux or Heartburn

Eat small meals and chew your food slowly. Do not lie down immediately after a meal; rather, sit upright for 1 to 2 hours after eating. Avoid spicy and fatty foods. Avoid caffeine. Do not chew gum. Do not wear tight waistbands. Avoid eating a large meal right before going to bed.

Constipation

Boost your fiber intake by eating lots of fresh fruits and vegetables, whole grain breads and cereals. Drink plenty of fluids. Tea, hot lemon water and juices such as prune juice are helpful. Stay physically active. Consider taking a short walk after meals. Go to the bathroom when you first feel the need.

Low Energy Levels

Eat a well-balanced diet consisting of regular meals and snacks. Try not to go more than 3 or 4 hours without eating. Stay well hydrated. Don't overexert yourself. Rest when you feel tired and consider going to bed an hour earlier than usual.

Eating for Energy
Sample Meals and Snacks

All of the following snacks provide between 200 and 300 calories.

- A peanut butter and jam sandwich on whole wheat bread and a glass of milk or soy milk.
- 8 whole grain crackers with cheddar cheese and a tart apple, such as Granny Smith.
- An energy bar, preferably made of natural ingredients, containing protein and carbohydrate with ½ cup fruit juice (try cranberry or apricot for a change) and a glass of water.
- ¾ cup yogurt with 1 cup fruit salad and a sprinkling of chopped, toasted almonds. Mangos, kiwi fruit, citrus fruits and berries are colorful and nutritious additions to a fruit salad.
- A smoothie made with 1/3 cup soft or dessert-style tofu, ½ cup milk or soy milk, 1 frozen banana, ½ cup fruit juice (orange juice works well) and ice as desired for thickness.
- 3 slices lean turkey meat on rye bread with a glass of tomato juice and a celery stalk.
- 2 slices pizza made with minimal amounts of cheese and processed meat, and lots of vegetables.
- A cranberry oat muffin, a banana and a steamed soy milk.

Sample Menu

Use this one-day sample menu as a guideline only. Exact portions of food needed will vary based on your weight, appetite and exercise level. Always remember to "cross-train" your diet by eating different meals and snacks to maximize your nutrient intake. Aim to eat 3 meals a day containing both protein (meat, meat alternatives and/or dairy foods) and carbohydrate (fruits, vegetables and whole grains) together with a glass of water for hydration. Choose quality snacks that taste good while providing maximum nourishment.

Breakfast

- 1 cup oatmeal or cream of wheat made with ¾ cup milk topped with ½ cup sautéed apples, ¼ cup toasted almonds, walnuts or pecans, 1 or 2 tablespoons raisins and a sprinkle of cinnamon.
- 1 cup fresh, calcium-fortified orange juice.
- Glass of water.

Snack

- 1 small container fruit-flavored yogurt with a sliced fresh peach or nectarine.
- Glass of water.

Lunch

- ½ can tuna mixed with ½ cup chopped red and yellow peppers, low-fat mayonnaise and seasonings inside a whole wheat pita pocket. Tuck in a few leaves of green leaf lettuce.
- 1 cup squash and vegetable soup.
- Glass of milk.
- Glass of water.

Snack

- 1 cup steamed milk or soy milk.
- 1 homemade or high quality oatmeal-raisin cookie or muffin.
- Glass of water.

Dinner

- 1 cup spinach salad made of fresh spinach and mushrooms.
- 4 or 5 ounces chicken breast stir-fried with 1½ cups assorted vegetables such as broccoli, carrots and green beans. Season with sesame oil and low-sodium sauces.
- 1 cup whole grain pasta or rice.
- Glass of water.

Notes

- If you are taking vitamins, take them with meals for maximum absorption.
- If you are vegetarian, substitute soy-based milk products for dairy in the above meal plan. At lunch, use a combination of beans such as kidney beans and chickpeas in place of tuna in the pita. For dinner, use firm tofu or a soy-based meat substitute in place of chicken in the stir-fry.

This meal plan supplies approximately 2400 calories, 50% carbohydrate, 25% protein and 25% fat. It meets the requirements for all nutrients including 16 mg of iron and 1600 mg of calcium.

Preconception Guidelines: Preparing for Pregnancy

As you prepare your body for conception, you may consider making important lifestyle changes during the year prior to conceiving. These can and should include quitting smoking, discontinuing alcohol and beginning an exercise program. Improving your fitness is one of the easiest and cheapest means to support a healthy pregnancy and healthy child.

Most women already know that a simple intervention like taking folic acid prior to conception can make their pregnancy a healthier one. But what about exercise? It has already been demonstrated that a woman who is active before her pregnancy receives the most benefit from a pregnancy exercise program. Furthermore, current studies indicate that exercise may in fact improve fertility. Encouraging fitness in the preconception stage is prudent in women of reproductive age.

If you already exercise regularly, you don't need to make any modifications during the preconception period unless fertility issues present themselves. If you are inactive, a moderate program including cardiovascular, strength (functional) and flexibility components should be started. The program should progress slowly with conservative increases in intensity, duration and frequency of exercise. Be aware that it takes the body approximately 4 to 6 weeks to adapt to a training program, and during that time it may be difficult to conceive. Ideally you would conceive once the fitness program is firmly established, approximately 3 months after beginning a new program.

Infertility and Exercise

The human body is an amazing machine that, when trained properly, functions ideally. Unfortunately, when over- or under-trained, the body often fails to perform. Pregnancy is the result of a complex series of hormonal interactions that can be affected by under-training, over-training and many other types of stress. In fact, any type of stress (nutritional, physical or physiological) may be enough to cause infertility problems in women.

For women who are too thin, due to either strict dieting or excessive exercise, these extreme behaviors are often the cause of their infertility (Bullen & Skrinar, 1984). Gaining weight or reducing the volume of exercise may help to reverse infertility. If a woman is overweight, obesity can exacerbate infertility. One study showed that weight loss alone can reverse infertility, in some cases. Weight loss does reduce the rate of miscarriage and improves the success of fertility treatment (Clark, Thornley & Tomlinson, 1998).

The George Washington University Center for Integrative Medicine believes some types of infertility are caused by a combination of several negative health behaviors, many of which can affect body weight. The Center promotes a focus on healthy eating, exercise and stress reduction as a means to eliminate infertility problems. Any time the body undergoes a radical change, infertility can be possible; therefore diet and exercise programs started preconception should begin and progress slowly so as not to exacerbate infertility issues.

Fit to Conceive 8-Week Walking Workout

In preparation for walking a 5-km event

This program consists of two parts, each with four separate weeks, for a total of eight weeks. Before beginning this or any other exercise program you should consult your physician or caregiver.

Adhere to the following guidelines:

- Don't become dehydrated. Drink 8 to 10 glasses of water daily.
- Don't overheat. Wear layered clothing and remove as needed.
- Don't over-train. Follow the program and listen to your body.
- Don't get overtired or exhausted. Walk on alternate days and take it easy if you are lacking energy.

Finding Your Fitness Level

Beginner: You are sedentary or never have been active on a consistent basis (exercising at least two times a week for a period of three months or more). Goal: Walk 5 km in 60 minutes plus.

Intermediate: You have been active at least two to three days per week for three months or more. You are able to power walk at least 30 minutes non-stop. Goal: Walk 5 km in 45 minutes plus.

Aerobic/Cardio Concerns

Terrain: Avoid slippery conditions, steep uphills which may tempt you to push your intensity level too far, and downhills because of the increased weight on your joints.

Intensity: Most people are familiar with taking and monitoring their heart rate during and after exercise. For effective training and efficient recovery, it is important to work within your target heart rate. Judging your rate of perceived exertion (RPE) is an ideal way of determining how hard you are working. Fit to Deliver uses the 10-point Borg scale, or talk test, in determining perceived exertion. During your walks you should easily be able to carry on a conversation; this would put you between 3 and 6 on the Borg scale, which is a good threshold for a moderate workout. If you can sing while you're walking you may want to pick up the pace a bit, and if you can't talk at all then you should take it down a notch. The benefit of using the RPE is that on a good day you can have a pretty brisk walk and still be within your limit of perceived exertion.

Training Tip: Power walking or running can be hard on your body, particularly your tendons and ligaments. Begin slowly and allow your body's tissues to adapt to the

NOTE

An 8- to 10-minute walk is equivalent to walking around the block.

	Duration of Walk (min.)	RPE	Total Workout Time[1]			Type of Walk	Duration of Walk (min.)	RPE	Total Workout Time[1]
BEGINNER					**INTERMEDIATE**				
Week 1					Week 1				
Day 1	10	3	20–25		Day 1	Power walk	25	4–5	35–40
Day 2	15	3	25–30		Day 2	Power walk	25	5	35–40
Day 3	10	3	20–25		Day 3	LSD[2]	30	5	40–45
Week 2					Week 2				
Day 1	15	3	25–30		Day 1	Power walk	30	4–6	40–45
Day 2	20	4	30–35		Day 2	Power walk	30	6	40–45
Day 3	15	3	25–30		Day 3	LSD	35	5	45–50
Week 3					Week 3				
Day 1	20	3	30–35		Day 1	Power walk	35	4–6	45–50
Day 2	25	3	35–40		Day 2	Power walk	35	6	45–50
Day 3	20	3	30–35		Day 3	LSD	40	5	50–55
Week 4 (Recovery)					Week 4 (Recovery)				
Day 1	15	3	25–30		Day 1	Power walk	30	5	40–45
Day 2	20	4	30–35		Day 2	Power walk	30	5	40–45
Day 3	15	3	25–30		Day 3	LSD	40	4–5	50–55
Week 5					Week 5				
Day 1	20	4	30–35		Day 1	Change of pace[3]	35	5–6	45–50
Day 2	25	3	35–40		Day 2	Power walk	35	5	45–50
Day 3	20	3	30–35		Day 3	LSD	45	4–5	50–55
Week 6					Week 6				
Day 1	25	4	35–40		Day 1	Change of pace	40	5–6	50–55
Day 2	30	3	40–45		Day 2	Power Walk	40	6	50–55
Day 3	25	3	35–40		Day 3	LSD	50	5	60–65
Week 7					Week 7				
Day 1	30	4	40–45		Day 1	Change of pace	45	5–6	55–60
Day 2	35	4	45–50		Day 2	Power Walk	40	6	50–55
Day 3	30	3	40–45		Day 3	LSD	55	5	60–65
Week 8 (Taper)					Week (Taper)				
Day 1	25	3	35–40		Day 1	Power walk	40	5	50–55
Day 2	30	3	40–45		Day 2	Power walk	40	5	50–55
Day 3	25	3	35–40		Day 3	LSD	50	4–5	60–65

[1] Total workout time includes warm-up and cooldown.
[2] LSD—Long slow distance.
[3] Change of pace power walk.

stresses. Remember to take into account the changes in your weight and center of gravity. You should do a slow walk into and out of your workout to allow a proper warm-up and cooldown.

Sample change of pace power walk

- Increase pace for 1 min, decrease to original pace for 4 min.
- Increase pace for 2 min, decrease to original pace for 4 min.
- Increase pace for 30 secs, decrease to original pace for 4 min.
- Increase pace for 1 min, decrease to original pace for 4 min, etc.

This is only a sample change of pace workout. Every change of pace power walk that you do will be different, based on your feelings and energy level that day. Always remember to listen to your body.

Cross-Training Techniques

If the weather is poor you may want to bring your workout indoors onto some cardio equipment to maintain your fitness level. These sample workouts are suitable for all fitness levels. If you are a beginner start

	Cardio Equipment	Duration	RPE
1a	Elliptical trainer	10 min.	3–6
1b	Treadmill	10 min.	3–5
1c	Stairclimber	10 min.	3–5
2a	Stairclimber	15 min.	3–5
2b	Elliptical trainer	10 min.	4–6
3a	Treadmill	15 min.	4–6
3b	Stairclimber	10 min.	4–6

slowly, doing only 10 minutes at a time on one piece of equipment (for example, 1a only). If you are intermediate or advanced you can complete the entire sample workout on more than one piece of equipment (for example, 1a, b, c) as a substitute for any of the power walking workouts. Before beginning your workout ensure a good dynamic warm-up (see chapter 5) and a proper cooldown.

Check the Borg scale for the RPE (rate of perceived exertion).

Pre-Conception Nutrition
It's Never too Early to Think About Healthy Eating
by Patricia Chuey

You've started trying to have a baby or recently found out you that you are pregnant. How wonderful! Congratulations! This is probably a key time in your life when your interest in eating well will be the strongest. As any responsible parent would want to do, you likely feel compelled to eat the most nourishing foods you can. Of course you don't have to be perfect. There are many barriers to healthy eating, including a lack of time, lack of energy and even conflicting messages on what is the best approach. These and other factors can make it tough to eat well all of the time. When you're pregnant or even while trying to get pregnant, it can also seem like everyone is giving you eating advice whether you want it or not. Ultimately you have to do what makes sense to you, within a few basic guidelines, to ensure you are getting all of the calories and nutrients you need to keep your energy level up and support your growing baby. If you follow the 80-20 rule of healthy eating and can honestly say you're eating well at least 80% of the time, you're doing great. It's okay to leave some room for leeway or special treats (20% of the time). And besides, you'll likely have some cravings that make it impossible for you to eat perfectly. In addition to an overall well-balanced diet consisting of foods from all food groups, you'll want to focus closely on a few key nutrients of special importance during pregnancy.

If you are planning on becoming pregnant, there are a few things you can do prior to conception to have the best pregnancy outcome. It is very important to take folic acid supplements (also called folate or folacin) for at least three months prior to conception. Experts recommend that all women of childbearing age and who are sexually active take 0.4 milligrams (4 micrograms) of folic acid a day. Folic acid is a B vitamin that is very important in the development of the baby's spinal cord, which occurs within the first four weeks of pregnancy (many women do not even realize that they are pregnant at this time). It helps to prevent neural tube defects, the most common being spina bifida in which the spinal cord does not close properly. Folic acid is abundant in many foods including green leafy vegetables (think "foliage"), oranges, orange juice, legumes, lentils, broccoli and other vegetables.

Before conception, it is also important to work on staying well nourished and to have good iron stores. (Your doctor can check your iron stores for you.) Low iron stores can result from avoiding animal protein without making appropriate substitutions or not eating enough calories overall. Iron is found in lean beef, clams, the dark meat of poultry, fish, enriched cereals, cream of

wheat, whole grains, beans and lentils, tofu, many soy foods and dark green vegetables. Iron absorption is enhanced when iron-rich foods are consumed with a source of vitamin C such as vegetables, fruit or fruit juice. If your eating habits are inconsistent and you struggle to eat enough volume or enough healthy foods, consider starting a prenatal supplement prior to conception. Keep in mind that supplements are just that —a *supplement* and not a *replacement* for healthy eating habits.

Work at maintaining an optimum weight for your size before conception as being overweight or underweight can affect your pregnancy. Talk to your doctor about your body mass index prior to getting pregnant. Body mass index (or BMI) is a better measure of whether you are in a healthy weight range for your height than simply using a rigid height-weight table. A healthy BMI is between 20 and 25. In addition to a healthy BMI, a healthy weight for you is one where you feel energetic, have a healthy immune system, don't get sick very often and feel comfortable. Healthy bodies come in many different shapes and sizes, even at the same weight.

A BMI above 27 is associated with health risks including heart disease, diabetes, cancer, sleep disorders and other concerns. Being significantly overweight can also contribute to infertility or a higher-risk pregnancy.

Being underweight at the time of conception can also pose health risks. It too can contribute to infertility. Risk for anemia (a lack of iron), heart problems and certain cancers can also be higher for the underweight person.

For good health overall, a balanced diet—high in fiber from fresh vegetables, fruits and whole grains—is recommended. A high-fiber diet assists in weight management and regularity, and is a factor in the prevention of diabetes and obesity. Unfortunately, advances in technology and consumers' increased desire for portable foods that are easy to eat on the run have led to the availability of more processed and refined foods. These foods often have had the fiber removed or had little fiber to begin with. Higher fiber wholesome foods have a lower glycemic index. (Glycemic index refers to the speed at which a food converts into sugar or energy when it enters the bloodstream.) Lower glycemic index foods include whole grains and brown rice, legumes, nuts, dairy products and many vegetables, among others. Higher glycemic index foods include white bread, white rice, refined cereals, high starch vegetables like carrots and potatoes, and foods high in sugar like soda pop, dessert and most candies. Eating lower glycemic index foods together with a

healthy lifestyle, including exercise, can help control blood sugar and energy levels. New research is suggesting that this style of eating may even be important in managing weight gain for mom and baby during pregnancy. An unbalanced diet (including high glycemic index foods) that keeps blood sugar levels high may result in more weight gain for mom, a bigger baby and a greater risk of diabetes.

In addition to making good food choices, before conception, look at your overall lifestyle habits. Aim to stay active with a regular, energizing exercise program. If you are smoker, pre-conception is the time to think about quitting. If you have concerns about alcohol use or other adjustments to make upon getting pregnant, talk to your doctor or a registered dietitian.

Lastly, before getting pregnant is not too soon to begin thinking about how you will feed your baby. This is a good time to begin discussing any questions you may have about breastfeeding or bottle-feeding with your healthcare team.

Selected References and Resources

American College of Obstetricians and Gynecologists (ACOG) Committee Opinion: Exercise during pregnancy and the postpartum period. *Obstetrics and Gynecology* 171–173, Jan. 2002.

Anderson, Bob. *Stretching.* Bolinas, CA: Shelter Publications, 1991.

Bo, Kari. Pelvic Floor Muscle Exercises. In *The Urinary Sphincter,* edited by J. Corcos and E. Schick. New York: Marcel Decker, Inc., 2001:443–457.

Bullen, B.A., G.S. Skrinar, and I.Z. Beitins, et al. Endurance training effects on plasma hormonal responsiveness and sex hormone excretion. *Journal of Applied Physiology* 56(6):1453–1463, June 1984.

Bullen, B., G. Skrinar, and I. Beitins, et al. Induction of menstrual disorders by strenuous exercise in untrained women. *New England Journal of Medicine* 312:1349–1353, 1985.

Canadian Academy of Sports Medicine. www.casm-acms.org.

Canadian Society for Exercise Physiology (CSEP). PARmed-X form available online at www.csep.ca.

Clapp III, James F., M.D. *Exercising Through your Pregnancy.* Omaha, Nebraska: Addicus Books, 2002.

Clapp, J.F. Morphometric and neurodevelopmental outcome at age five years of the offspring of women who continued to exercise regularly throughout pregnancy. *Pediatrics* 129(6), 856–63, Dec. 1996.

Clapp, J.F. The effects of maternal exercise on early pregnancy outcome. *American Journal of Obstetrics and Gynecology* 161(6 Pt 1), 1453–1457, Dec. 1989.

Clark, A., B. Thornley, and L. Tomlinson, et al. Weight loss in obese infertile women results in improvement in reproductive outcome for all forms of fertility treatment. *Human Reproduction* 13(6):1502–1505, 1998.

Collings, C., C. Curet, and J. Mullin. Maternal and Fetal Responses to a Maternal Aerobic Exercise Program. *American Journal of Obstetrics and Gynecology* 145 (6), 702–707, 1983.

Hall, D., and D. Kaufmann. Effects of aerobic and strength conditioning on pregnancy outcomes. *American Journal of Obstetrics and Gynecology* 157(5), 1199–1203, 1987.

Jones, R. The pelvic floor. *Current Concepts of Pelvic Floor Muscle Rehabilitation—Orthopaedic Division Review* 17–19, Jan./Feb. 2002.

Kendall, Florence Peterson and Elizabeth Kendall McCreary. *Muscles: Testing and Function.* Philadelphia: Williams & Wilkins, 1993.

Kisner, Carolyn, and Lynn Allen Colby. *Therapeutic Exercise: Foundations and Techniques.* Philadelphia: F.A. Davis Company, 1990.

Lee, D. PostPartum Health for Moms. www.dianelee.ca/postpartum/.

McKechnie, Alex, and Rick Celebrini. Hard Core Strength: A Practical Application of Core Training for Rehabilitation of the Elite Athlete. Course notes. Vancouver, BC, April 2002.

Nordahl, Karen, and Carl Petersen, et al. *Fit to Deliver.* Vancouver, BC: Fit to Deliver International Inc., 2000.

Richardson, C.A., G.A. Jull, P.W. Hodges, and J. Hides. *Therapeutic Exercise for Spinal Segmental Stabilisation in Low Back Pain.* Edinburgh: Churchill Livingstone, 1999.

Sapsford, R.R., P.W. Hodges, C.A. Richardson, D.H. Cooper, S.J. Markwell, and G.A. Jull, et al. Coactivation of the abdominal and pelvic floor muscles during voluntary exercises. *Neurourology and Urodynamics* 20:31–42, 2001.

Index

About the Authors

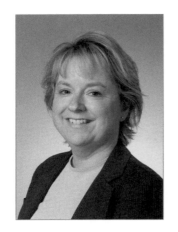

Karen Nordahl, MD

Karen Nordahl is a medical doctor who practices family medicine and obstetrics at the BC Women's Hospital in Vancouver. She received her medical degree from the University of British Columbia in 1989. She has an undergraduate degree in Kinesiology (Physiology) from Simon Fraser University in Burnaby, BC. Dr. Nordahl is head of the Burnaby Medical Association and is a clinical associate instructor at the University of British Columbia's Faculty of Medicine. Dr. Nordahl is on the editorial advisory boards of *Fit Pregnancy* and *Living Fit* magazines.

Early in her medical career, Dr. Nordahl discovered that there was very little authoritative information available for women who questioned whether to remain active during pregnancy. She began to research the subject, joining forces with renowned physical therapist and trainer Carl Petersen, to develop a prenatal and postpartum fitness program, self-published as *Fit to Deliver* in 2000. Renée Jeffreys joined the team in 2001, co-authoring this edition of *Fit to Deliver* as well as the "Fit to Deliver Certification Program" for fitness professionals. Dr. Nordahl's goal is to provide all women with the tools to exercise safely during pregnancy, and to make pregnancy both healthier and easier.

The authors offer courses for health and fitness professionals in Canada, the United States and Great Britain, using *Fit to Deliver* as an instruction manual. Fitness professionals in other countries around the world are also adopting the "Fit to Deliver" program for use with their clients.

Dr. Nordahl has been interviewed on radio and television, and featured in national and regional newspapers and magazines. She and the "Fit to Deliver" team also regularly contribute to *Urban Baby* magazine, and several websites including ivillage, WebMD and canoe.com.

Carl Petersen, BPE, BSc (PT)

Carl Petersen is a physical therapist and fitness coach. He completed his Bachelor of Physical Education degree in 1980 and his Bachelor of Science degree (Physical Therapy/Occupational Therapy) in 1983, both at the University of British Columbia.

Petersen is currently the director of high-performance training at his City Sports & Physiotherapy Clinics in Vancouver, BC. He works with World Cup skiers, professional tennis players and club-level athletes. During his time with the Canadian Alpine Ski Team, he coached and designed training programs for World Cup, Olympic and World Championship medalists. He was a member of Canada's medical team for three Winter Olympic Games, and was named Ski

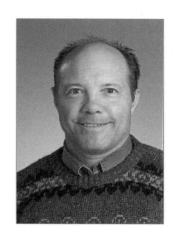

Canada's "Best of the Best Knee Physiotherapists" in 1998.

A frequent television guest and speaker at international conferences, Petersen is well known in the fields of physical therapy, physical and sports training, injury prevention and pregnancy fitness. He educates and assists other health professionals in teaching women about exercise and injury prevention during pregnancy. He is the author of the sports training books *Fit to Play Tennis* and *Fit to Ski*. He is a frequent contributor to consumer sports and fitness magazines and to professional journals.

Renée Minges Jeffreys, MSc

Renée Minges Jeffreys is an exercise physiologist and personal trainer. An avid runner, Jeffreys completed her first marathon in 1994 and went on to obtain several aerobics and personal training certifications. These include ACSM Health & Fitness Instructor, ACE Personal Trainer and Clinical Exercise Specialist, AEA Water Aerobics Instructor, AFAA Land Aerobics Instructor, USATF Level One Track and Field Coach, and American Red Cross Health and Safety Instructor. She is also a member of the American College of Sports Medicine (ACSM).

A passion for women's health and fitness led to graduate school at George Washington University in Washington, DC where Jeffreys interned with James F. Clapp III, MD, an expert on prenatal fitness. She received her masters degree in exercise science, and her thesis focused on prenatal fitness

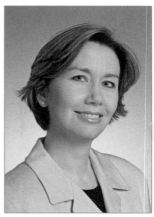

programs and their effect on labor, delivery, physical discomfort and maternal self-esteem. Currently, she and Dr. Clapp are collaborating on a study investigating exercise in the supine position and its impact on uterine blood flow.

Jeffreys owns and operates Fitness for Women, LLC in Cincinnati, Ohio, which offers personal training, group classes and consulting services. She is also the exercise physiologist for the Holistic Health Center at St. Elizabeth Medical Center in Cincinnati. Jeffreys is an exercise advisor to *Fit Pregnancy* magazine.

Jeffreys and her husband Mark have two children. She maintained her fitness throughout both pregnancies.